Reflections

Endorsements

"This is a gripping story of life, healing, and the love that shines through it all. It is in life's exposed inner core that the magical transformation occurs during our final scene. It is there we make the sudden shifts between the revealing light and the invading shadow—the light inescapably insightful and precious.

Everything that had been pushed aside by fear and negligence, by ignorance and complacency, is invited back by Brian Hobbs who, with openness and candor, allows life to finally catch up to him. With incredible loyalty and insight into wholeness and healing, his wife Fia Hobbs navigates them both, in acceptance and in healing. Day by day, moment by moment, all the way to death's door, which perhaps needn't always divide us, they both stand in our presence as a universal teacher and guide.

The impact of Brian's healing at the end of his life leaves an unforgettable touch of hope and purpose, and a reminder of the finiteness that we all need to be reminded of to live in the here and now. My wish is for everyone to take part in this story that sheds light on the inescapably painful part of the totality of life."

—Marie Bergman
Swedish singer-songwriter, therapist.

"Through Brian and Fia's writing I have followed along on their difficult journey and been uplifted by their fighting spirit, strength, wisdom and love for one another and for life itself. The text conveys not only emotion and reflection but guiding advice that can be of great help to many.

The book provides an intimate window into two experiences, one from a cancer patient's perspective and the other through the eyes of a loved one and caregiver. Never before have I encountered a book where there was such an intimate and heartfelt exchange between two voices as this one."

—**Stig Hanno**
Chairman of the patient and caregiver
advisory board of Swedish RCC, Regional Cancer Center
Stockholm/Gotland.

"A truly inspirational book on life and death and having a purpose in life that will stay with you for a long time."

—**Kevin Harrington**, Original Shark on "Shark Tank",
Inventor of the Infomercial, Best Selling Author

"With heartfelt honesty, this book takes us on the roller coaster ride of having a cancer diagnosis in a most sensitive manner. Although it acknowledges the difficulties that are experienced by most patients and caregivers, it spares us the intimate details of treatments gone wrong, fears that consume us, and the mental and physical toll of caring for someone with cancer, as many books of this nature do. Instead, it focuses on how do we stay present? How do we remain hopeful? What important information has been learned that can be left behind that may help others on this cancer journey?

Written by a brilliantly poetic musician and his compassionate therapist wife, we feel the power of our thoughts on our well-being. We see the critical importance of support. We understand the significance of giving and receiving love…love of family, friends, nature, our universe… and how all of this impacts our physiology, our life, our health, RIGHT NOW, regardless if we are currently ill or well.

Every cancer journey is personal. We all have something to gain from each other's experiences if we are privileged enough to be invited in. This is your invitation."

—**Karen Smith Simonton**, Executive Director,
Simonton Cancer Center

Reflections

A Story of HOPE, HEALING, Facing FEARS, and Finding PURPOSE

Brian & Fia Hobbs

NEW YORK

LONDON • NASHVILLE • MELBOURNE • VANCOUVER

Reflections

A Story of HOPE, HEALING, Facing FEARS, and Finding PURPOSE

Published in New York, New York, by Morgan James Publishing. Morgan James is a trademark of Morgan James, LLC. www.MorganJamesPublishing.com

ISBN 978-1-64279-706-0 paperback
ISBN 978-1-64279-707-7 eBook
Library of Congress Control Number: 2019908975

Cover Design by:
Chris Treccani
www.3dogcreative.net

Interior Design by:
Bonnie Bushman
The Whole Caboodle Graphic Design

Front Cover Photo:
John Jacobsson

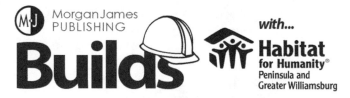

Morgan James is a proud partner of Habitat for Humanity Peninsula and Greater Williamsburg. Partners in building since 2006.

Get involved today! Visit
www.MorganJamesBuilds.com

Dedication

This book is dedicated to my sons,
Adam and Jeremy Hobbs.
I am so thankful for having you
in my life and for your support.
For you Brian, always present with
your songs and lyrics and in our hearts.
Much Love!
Fia Hobbs

Table of Contents

Foreword by Dr Saupe

For more than 30 years, the disease called cancer have been the main subject of my studies of life-sciences and my challenging companion as a seeker for better cancer therapies.

It started with the diagnosis of my mother when I was a student in my third year of medical school, continued with her fast progressing breast cancer and her death in my arms when she was 54. It has been the main diagnosis of the patients who see me in my life as a medical doctor ever since.

The book *Reflections* touched my heart on every page when I read it. It brought back memories from the time I took care of my mother during the last three months of her life and of many patients and their relatives in whose treatment of late stage cancer I was involved. From all these experiences I can say that this book tells us about an important part of our life that we normally do not talk so much about: the chapter of our life when dying and death comes closer. The book reflects on the meaning of that in a very personal, poetic, honest and philosophical way, all at the same time.

This book is a powerful and important aid for the reader because of three factors:

First, it can help everyone who is in a situation like Brian's, one of the two main characters, confronted with a non-curable disease and the time that is left to live while the disease relentlessly takes over. Brian's open-hearted way of letting us come into his intimate life full of struggle, desperation, gratefulness and deep trust in a divine plan can be a remedy for every cancer patient. In his poems, Brian expresses it better than any academic or psychological description could ever do. It also shows the other side of the drama, beyond the weakening of the body: the insights and change of consciousness that we can get from the existential crisis cancer confronts us with.

Second, it has one simple and fundamental message above all: love is what we live for and what is most important when our lives are at stake.

And third, because it takes us by the hand in a day-to-day practical introduction into the healthy mindset called mindfulness-awareness. It does this through the reflections of Brian's wife Fia's insightful, non-judgmental, accepting and unconditionally loving attitude. This can be a remedy for everyone who lives with a loved one who is in Brian's situation.

I hope this book reaches out to the many, many people who are in a similar situation, to cancer patients, spouses, family members, nurses, medical doctors and friends of those who are challenged with cancer. The insights of this book can make our lives easier, more conscious, more peaceful and more loving.

Dr Henning Saupe

Acknowledgements

I would like to thank my son Adam Hobbs for his invaluable assistance in editing this book. My son Jeremy for helping out so much during Brian's illness. I also want to thank my sister for being supportive in so many ways.

A special thank you to Brian's family for their love and support and who helped us out financially, and to his sister who started a GoFundMe to pay for treatments.

I also want to thank everyone who helped us out in our most difficult time, you made a world of difference to Brian and me. To mention you all would fill a book on its own.

A heartfelt thank you to all!

Fia Hobbs

Prologue

Brian Hobbs started to write about his challenge facing late stage cancer as a way of handling his own fears and to inspire others dealing with a serious illness.

This book is based on the blog he wrote during the seven months from his diagnosis to his death on February 8, 2018. The blog became a huge inspiration to many people and he received an astounding response.

He also wanted me to write from my perspective as a wife and caregiver, as well as his counseling therapist. It is a role I know well, mainly from my work but also from having lost many friends to cancer. I was both his wife and psychological support and over the months, as he grew in spirituality, we had long conversations about life and death. Brian wanted to spread his message and was hoping in the early days that he could speak to people about finding purpose in life whatever they were up against, including facing death. He became passionate about helping people get over the fears that stop so many of us, something that he himself had struggled with for most of his life.

Unfortunately he was not able to fulfill the idea of public speaking but he did become a huge inspiration through his blog, especially to his singer-songwriter students. We were both overwhelmed by the response and he was lucky to find out while he was still alive that he had been an inspiration to many people over the years, without even being aware of it. He just followed his passion.

Fia Hobbs

The Blog

My name is Brian Hobbs and I am a cancer patient.

I just had a major operation to remove one of my kidneys and the large tumor that was attached to it. Won't bore you with the details, the heading pretty much says it.

When you're somewhat incapacitated, as I have been most of this summer, you have plenty of time to ponder. I've spent a lot of time going to my "happy places" (revisiting people I have loved and places that have brought me joy). I also realized how thankful I am for so much.

My Happy Places
August 23, 2017

*M*y "happy places" consist of many childhood memories; so please bear with me while I list a few.

Staying with my Grandma Hobbs and being greeted with an ice-cold "Co-cola" (that was her way of pronouncing it). Her giving me a quarter and walking down to Mr. Paul's store on Creek Road where I could get an orange popsicle, football, baseball or Batman cards, Sweet Tarts and Bazooka Joe bubble gum.

Staying with my Grandma and Granddaddy Meads and helping him in his garden, enjoying a dinner (read lunch…in the south at that time the daily meals consisted of breakfast, dinner and supper) with fried chicken, boiled greens and potatoes, cornbread, sweet tea, homemade biscuits, and if I was lucky, a piece of Grandma's chocolate cake. Granddaddy always had peppermint chewing gum and we'd chew that after dinner and sit out in the swing in summer.

Visiting my father at Culpepper Motor Company on Elizabeth St. and looking at the new cars in the showroom. I especially loved

Christmastime because there was a big aluminum tree there and a life-size Santa sitting in one of the chairs.

Friday nights at Granddaddy and Grandma Meads' when most of my aunts, uncles and cousins came over and we heard stories from long ago out on the front porch with background sounds provided by frogs and crickets and the occasional car riding down Thunder Road with the radio on and windows down. My cousins and I played until we were exhausted and covered in sweat. That's when we'd come in and get a drink of cold water from a green pitcher filled with rainwater from inside my grandmother's ancient Frigidaire.

Weekends at my parents' place down on the Albemarle Sound where my imagination ran wild with images of pirates, Indians, damsels in distress and whatever other images I conjured up from the books I read. My mother would cook fried potatoes and green beans and daddy would grill burgers or pork chops. It was heavenly! When I got older I would drive down there alone with my high-school girlfriend (although "alone" is probably not the correct term). As live, walking contraceptives, we were always accompanied by my sister and at least 2-3 of my girlfriend's younger siblings. It worked.

Saturday mornings when my mother and I were home alone and we would listen to music (an awful lot of Gershwin) while we cleaned.

My father teaching me to play golf.

Band trips…anything to do with the band.

Soft ice-cream from Nu-Quality in the summer.

Stopping in to see Grandma and Granddaddy Hobbs after church on Sunday nights and getting powdered donuts, another Co-cola and maybe a slice of plain cake with white icing.

Hearing my mother play piano or organ at church.

Christmas pageants.

Church picnics. Dinner on the grounds.

My parents taking me to Peter Nero concerts in Norfolk…

There are many other people and places that I have visited but that's enough for now. In addition to visiting my "happy places" I also started counting my blessings:

A devoted wife who has been with me through this whole ordeal, and in addition to taking excellent care of me, has also dealt with all the practicalities of insurance, doctors, phone calls, as well as my own ups and downs, etc.

My two boys, who have taken time out from their lives to help out at home and also kept me laughing.

A mother and father who are still there for me in every way.

A sister who has been extremely supportive and helped my mother and father help me.

Family on both sides of the Atlantic who have helped out and kept me in their thoughts and prayers.

Friends who have offered to help in any way they can, along with colleagues and former students who have showered me with love and good thoughts.

My main songwriting collaborators who continue to check in and inspire me. (I'm horribly afraid that one day they will find out they don't need me).

The fact that I made it through major surgery and still ended up on this side of the dirt.

The fact that after only 3 weeks I'm relatively mobile and feeling as good as could be expected.

That I can listen to music again and that it moves me more than ever.

That I can see beauty and find joy where I never saw it before.

That "petty bulls***", which somehow was incorrectly filed under "IMPORTANT" in my life has now been refiled under "PETTY BULLS***—deal with this later".

All in all, I'm happy. Of course I wish I didn't have cancer and I still don't know what the outcome will be but I'm positive, thoughtful and thankful. And my advice to everyone is this: take your moments and create "happy places" for yourself and people you love. Never forget that the most insignificant things you do (like giving someone a quarter to buy an orange popsicle on a hot summer day, or just spending time with someone) can be a lifetime memory for them. And don't be afraid to turn around and look your mortality in the face. It's the best way to remind yourself to keep "petty bulls***" in the right file. And most importantly, love each other and be kind.

Thanks for reading and please check out the rest of my site. And if you want to start being especially kind...download or stream my album, GENESIS OF WHO I AM.

Best, Brian

The Diagnosis

A background

On July 17, 2017 I was diagnosed with kidney cancer. I had a 12 centimeter tumor on my left kidney. An operation was planned immediately but it had already metastasized to the liver. I don't think the seriousness hit me until much later. I was more fascinated by the size of the tumor on my kidney. It wasn't until much later that I realized that it was a death sentence. It changed my life obviously. I'm still not sure I realized the gravity of the situation until I spoke with the oncologist. You can see that in my first blog entry. This was written before meeting with the oncologist.

I had had thyroid cancer seven years earlier and that was a walk in the park. This cancer would not be. It was aggressive and nasty. I was preparing for the operation not thinking about the disease. I felt the operation would clear the cancer. How naive I was. I gradually realized that I had a very serious disease that could kill me.

My wife was with me the whole time, giving strength and guiding me. Like I wrote, I was naive and still had no idea what I was up against. That naïveté came crashing down around me over the next few months.

I guess it hit me hardest when my doctor put a number on things. I was told that with treatment I could expect an average survival rate of 22 months. I was then given information about the drug, Sutent. After looking at the literature with my wife we both decided the side effects took away all quality of life and opted out. We did agree to start a second level of treatment with Votrient. I ended up taking the drug for six days.

Before, I had been able to sit and walk a little but the treatment totally incapacitated me. It took more than a week to recover from the effects of the drug. After that, Karolinska hospital cut me loose and I was placed in palliative care, which meant that as far as any recovery was concerned I was on my own.

Fia's Reflections

I knew from the start that it was a tough diagnosis. I decided not to let Brian know just how serious it was as I feared he would have given up immediately and not even wanted to go through with the surgery if he knew.

Brian had thyroid cancer back in 2010 and although he describes it as a walk in the park, and it was in comparison to the kidney cancer, it still shook him to the core. About six months after the operation there was a psychological backlash that proved to be a struggle for him. I thought the first cancer, being a wake-up call, would have inspired Brian to make more changes to his lifestyle but it lasted only about six months before he returned to his old habits of too much candy, bad diet, no exercise and an overload of work.

I have seen the same thing happen in others as I work with cancer patients and their families as a counseling therapist. It shakes you and makes you realize that your life has an expiration date and how we treat our bodies affects our quality of life.

Being human we tend to fall back into old habits once the dust has settled; we forget the importance of a healthy lifestyle, claiming that you cannot live your life being fearful of recurrence. You just want to get on with life again and that is what Brian did.

Looking Back into the Lens

August 29, 2017

I have an old camera sitting in my writing space that I found in my parents' attic; a Kodak Duaflex II. I've had this camera for years but never really thought about it other than as an adornment and dust catcher on my bookshelf. But I can be a little obsessive about things once I do start thinking about them so I picked it up and looked through the viewfinder. Intrigued, I started a little online research and found that it was produced between 1950 and 1954 and originally sold for around 22 dollars. You looked into the viewfinder and focused on your subject by holding it in front of you at waist level. I'm sure that many of the photos I have looked at in my parents' old albums were taken with this camera.

As I was looking at it and reading about it I imagined what a wondrous thing it would be to look into the lens, through the camera and back in time into the mind and soul of everyone who'd ever taken a photo or been photographed with that camera. I imagined looking into my father or mother's mind and seeing the world through their eyes as newlyweds in 1955; young, naive, and hopeful. I saw the posed and spontaneous photos of their friends and relatives, many now departed

7

from this life, whose images were captured by this tiny camera. I saw youth and joy. Even though the images were black & white I saw the colors of spring and summer, the flowery dresses and two-tone shoes, azaleas in blossom, Easter Sunday, men with flowers in their lapels, weddings and bouquets, women in hats, old relatives that died before I was born, younger versions of people in my life that I came to love, images of them when the world was at their feet, before disease, disappointment and heartbreak changed them, before the full impact of life and living punched them in the face and left them bruised and scarred.

And all this made me remember talking to an uncle of mine shortly before he died. He was beaten down by debt and bad health, living with a person that was his wife in name only…her mind was gone and she sat in the corner in a rocking chair staring out from blank and hollow eyes. By some grace of God she sat there with a permanent smile, sometimes gently talking to herself. I had gone over to their house one morning with my mother when she was bringing them breakfast. While my mother fed my aunt I sat in the kitchen across from my uncle. With tears in his eyes he said: "Son, I never thought my life would end up like this."

And in that one sentence I realized why God or the Universe never lets us see the future. It was hard for me to hold back the tears. Is there a response to such a thing?

But I have always been an observer and a searcher, so in my mind I snapped a photo. Even though it is painful to look at; his wizened, blemished face and sad, far-away looking eyes; the photo in my mind's eye captured all the beauty and pain of this life; the love, anguish, regret and joy of living.

Photos are memories captured on paper or reproduced as a set of digits. Memories are photos in the mind; places we've been, people we've loved, moments we've shared, good times and hard times, all adding up to the sum of our existence. But our existence is so much more than the way we leave this life.

I wish that I had had the Duaflex camera with me that morning at my uncle's house. I would have asked him to look back into the lens and I would have let him see and relive some of his happy moments. It's taken me a while to gain even a modicum of understanding of the whats and whys of this life, but I think I have learned that it's not about where you are at the end of it, but it's more about the journey of getting there.

No matter what life throws our way I hope we all have a Duaflex camera in our mind and that we can look back into the lens and sometimes see ourselves as young, naive and hopeful; when we had the whole world at our feet.

Here Is Another Day, What Are You Going to Do with It?

September 2, 2017

*T*hat is the question I woke up with echoing inside my head after going back to bed this morning. I had awakened about 2 hours earlier with the mantra of "I'm going to die".

In hindsight, "I'm going to die" seems ludicrous. Of course I am! Everyone is! But upon my first wake up I talked to my wife, a surprisingly smart woman even though she married me. We had talked about acceptance (not resignation or giving up) and that old standby of taking it one day at a time. And as I'm writing this I'm remembering one of my favorite lyrics "Tomorrow Doesn't Care" that I wrote with Leif Larsson that was performed by the LOST VAN GOGHS. I'll put the Spotify link to the song at the end of the post, but here are the lyrics:

TOMORROW DOESN'T CARE
You can plan your life away, always living on the run
Lose yourself in small details, never give your heart to anyone
Waiting for the moment to seize the perfect day

Hoping for atonement, throwing it away
You can't live in tomorrow
Building castles in the air
Don't you know this time is borrowed
And tomorrow doesn't care
And you can dream until you're blind, and keep collecting all your
  souvenirs
Tell yourself those pretty lies as you just fade away and disappear
Lost in discontentment, walking in a trance
Hiding your resentment, scared to take a chance
You can't live in tomorrow
Building castles in the air
Don't you know this time is borrowed
And tomorrow doesn't care
And it might not still be there
You can't live in tomorrow
Building castles in the air
Don't you know this time is borrowed
And tomorrow doesn't care
Don't you know this time is borrowed
And tomorrow doesn't care

I wrote that…so what the hell am I sitting there worrying about "I'm going to die, I'm going to die"?

Well, I went back to bed and slept off and on for a sweaty, uncomfortable two hours. And when I woke up it was like a fever had broken and I was looking around my room, thankful and thoughtful because I was hearing "Here is another day, what are you going to do with it?" instead of "I'm going to die".

So I ate breakfast and sat down at the computer and started writing this. And I'm sure there will be other days when I lapse into the fever of self-pity, but hopefully the fever will break again and I'll come out on the other side saying "Here is another day, what are you going to do with it?".

And here is the link to TOMORROW DOESN'T CARE: Spotify:track:655pnW8BeyTcZVjwGJv5dK

Fia's Reflections

On August 30 Brian had to go back to the hospital for severe pain in his abdomen. We thought it had something to do with the previous operation, so they gave him an x-ray and kept him over night. The day after they sent him to another hospital to meet his oncologist for the first time. She was not prepared to take him on and sent him back to the first hospital, who in their turn was done with him and could not help him any further. Brian was weak and tired and feeling like no one knew what to do with him so I took him home. This explained his mantra about going to die.

Brian has gone through a huge transformation after he got his cancer diagnosis in July 2017. He has started to contemplate life and death with an emphasis on life. Our talks are long and for the first time he is truly interested in what I have been working with for years, work that he never quite understood before. I guess a lot of people think that working with cancer patients must be depressing but that is far from the truth. I find it liberating to be able to cut to the chase and quickly discover what truly matters and from there work to improve the quality of life.

I am also thankful for the 30 years of mental training I have including qigong, meditation and mindfulness. It helps to keep me grounded and present in the now, especially when facing a situation that I don't know how or when it will end.

Our discussions take place in the morning when Brian wakes up as he has often had time to lie and reflect before I wake up. Also our afternoon talks in the healing room have become sacred for Brian, this is where he lets out all his worries in a safe environment. The healing room is situated in our house and it has a calm energy about it. This is where I have my work bench and give healing to Brian and where we talk.

It has been easier than I thought taking on the role as his professional therapist and we go deep into the mystery of life and death. When I go back to the role of being a wife, my training helps me to focus on the here and now. If I allow myself to look too far ahead it becomes too overwhelming. Together we take it one day at a time.

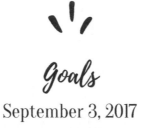

Goals

September 3, 2017

Live to see my sons graduate (in June 2018)—
See my family again (from the States)—check
Gain weight to at least 85 kilos—
Finish and release Impressions II, (my instrumental album)—check
Write to people and say what they mean to me—check
Finish *Dance Me into Forever*—

Fia's Reflections

Brian wrote a bucket list early on and these goals were on top of the list. He managed to fulfill three of them during the year and in total released five albums and one book about songwriting called The Craft of Creating. It was as if he let go of his fear of releasing albums that, in his mind, were not quite perfect. He put out Genesis of Who I Am, Reflections, Impressions II, The Independent Man (a musical) and Healing Purpose. The album Reflections quickly turned into a treasured album with some of his favorite singers and collaborators performing and playing. He was very proud of how everyone pulled together to get it finished. I cannot thank the people involved in the production enough for what they did!

I know that he was very pleased with his solo album Genesis of Who I Am, although he was scared when he released it in June 2017. He was not comfortable singing and after the release his voice started getting hoarse and weaker but at that time we still did not know that he had cancer. He thought it was due to his heart problems and that he was exhausted. He was waiting to get a new heart valve but time was dragging out.

A Face of False Bravado

September 6, 2017

Making jokes as the hangman puts the noose around your neck
Whistling in the dark
Trying hard to be the strong one
Feeling like you're the hoax
Because one day your facade crumbles
And you are that little boy again
Left alone on the carousel
And you want everything to stop, or fast forward
Or rewind
You want to be anywhere other than where you are now
Your silent curses and anger steal your strength
And you think of the ones you will leave behind
And you want the cleansing tears to flow
But they don't and you are surrounded by
Nothingness and the shells of every dry existence
You fear death, you long for it
For any peace, for a proper denouement to
Your story

Yesterday, a Good Day
September 8, 2017

I released myself from life and wrote my desires for my memorial service. And then without bargaining, I envisioned myself talking about my story, my healing, my beliefs. And in a most undramatic way God told me "OK, you will be healed".

I have already accepted my death so I have decided to believe. Maybe my story can help someone. I only know that I feel better and stronger, more positive, more ready to focus on living instead of focusing on not dying.

Fia's Reflections

We talk a lot about acceptance. It is a word that always comes up when I talk to anyone who is stuck in life or if someone has cancer or any other serious illness. How can you accept that you have cancer? Does it mean that you have to like it? Does it mean you have given in, given up on life?

Acceptance only means that you acknowledge where you are right now. No more, no less. You don't have to like it and you can even be angry for having it, but nevertheless it is there and you have to start with accepting the fact.

It is what you do after the acceptance that will lead you further to the next step, whatever that might be. Knowing that you will die regardless of whether you have cancer or not can be liberating. The only thing we know for sure is that we are born and somewhere down the line we die. In between is what we call life and what we choose to do with it is up to us. I think we are here to have experiences and to grow as human beings and with that comes happiness and sorrow. We cannot shut out the sad parts of life, they are part of the deal, just like being born and taking your first breath or the head over heels feeling of being in love.

Shifting your mind and thoughts from "I don't want to die" to "I am ready to live" has a profound impact on the way you will feel and move forward. In fear or in hope, it is a choice.

Small Kindnesses, Major Changes
September 10, 2017

I received a lovely bouquet of flowers yesterday from the wife of a friend. Now I don't know her that well, we've probably only met and socialized a few times, but I know she's a good person because I have seen the change in my friend over the last couple of years. He's calmer, happier and a lot more contented and I know that she has played a big role in that.

In her note she thanked me for the support and friendship I'd given her husband over the time we've been friends. The fact is this, my friend has given me probably twice the support I've given him, but I'm grateful for small kindnesses. Her gesture touched and moved me in a major way. And as I read her note a wave of thankfulness swept over me once again for all the people who have stopped by, sent messages, flowers and gifts, and called and kept me in their thoughts and prayers.

This disease I have is a hateful one, and I'm sure there are many people out there who can relate. But the amazing thing is that it has made me more thankful, thoughtful and aware, more filled with purpose than at any time in my life. It's like I found a hidden room filled with my purpose, my reasons for wanting to live. So I'm dusting them off and polishing them up because I will need them to be at their best to go up against my disease and win. In the beginning I had a pretty common, negative take on the whole situation; I didn't want to die. Through the small kindnesses I've turned it around and now my mantra is "I would rather focus on living than focus on NOT dying". Some people might think there's no difference but to me that's a major change in attitude.

I still don't know how my story is going to end (just like none of us do), but I am positive and hopeful and thankful; thankful that small kindnesses lead to major changes, and major changes give us our purpose. Thanks Anna!

Hope and Hurt

September 13, 2017

*T*hese are my thoughts from September 13. It's taken a couple of days to get them transferred from my notebook to the blog:
Hope is a powerful thing, but as my mother always told me, "where there's hope there's hurt". True; it goes up and down all the time. One minute it's total despair and the next immense gratitude and positivity.

That's how it started for me today. My demons came out in full force and threw everything they had at me. Fortunately, I have a wife who listens, understands and keeps me grounded. My demons had me wanting to die, had stolen all my hope during the night, but after admitting how scared, angry and hopeless I was and crying, really crying, for the first time since this ordeal began, it was like I had a catharsis. I don't know what it was, but during a treatment from my wife today I felt better. I was anxious to get off that table, I got strength from the music I was listening to…my music. It was like I rediscovered my purpose.

Tears come and sometimes they bring doubts and my demons drink the bitterness and grow strong again, but sometimes the tears are cleansing and open my eyes to being thankful and thoughtful once

21

again, and just like that Al Jarreau song, Mornin', I feel I can reach out my hand and touch the face of God. There's so much love and beauty in the world, and of course that's balanced with hate and ugliness.

I started my morning with despair and am now moving towards ending my day with hope. Will my demons come back in force? I'm sure they will, but right now I am going to wrap up in a quilt my mother made me that is filled with love and I am going to let myself be warmed by the divine sparks from all the people who love me and are keeping me in their thoughts and prayers. So…for now, I'll keep reaching out to touch the face of God. There are still many questions and I have found so few answers, but like my wife just said, "answers are overrated, it's the questions that are interesting".

Fia's Reflections

One of the most important things you can do is to hold a safe space for someone who is in despair and just listen to them. Just being there, not trying to come up with solutions or "cheering" them up. There is no use in trying to hide and sweep sadness under the rug, sooner or later it will always show up and come back with a vengeance. In our society we now give pills to people who suffer losses or go through minor depression. It is seen as abnormal to be unhappy or sad. There is a diagnosis for just about everything. I on the other hand think there is a lack of giving people time to heal and for someone to acknowledge what they are going through and just being there to listen and to provide a safe space for them to heal the pain.

The treatment Brian is talking about is a hyperthermia (heat) lamp I use for different kinds of pain in general (this helped him to be free of pain during his whole cancer diagnosis up until the very end when he could no longer get up on the treatment table). The treatment also involves healing and talking. It is a sacred hour for both of us and Brian feels free to ventilate everything that is on his mind and get it out while I am holding a safe space for him. My own safe space is my daily call to my sister, cuddling my dog and doing my mindfulness practice. That is all I have time for as I am with Brian 24/7. He gets worried when I have to leave even for an hour to get groceries or take the dog out, even though one of our sons is at home. Brian says he feels safe when I am at home as he knows I will deal with anything that can happen and I am glad I can give him that security and safe space.

Better Start to the Day Today

September 14, 2017

*B*etter start to the day today! Feeling positive but just want to get answers from the doctor and finalize my decision about treatment.

Fia's Reflections

On September 11 we went to the hospital to talk about possible treatment that could prolong Brian's life as there was no curative treatment. We talked to the nurse and got all our questions answered and the side effects were tremendous. We politely listened and told her that we would think about it.

The decision was easy. Brian wanted to be "healthy" for as long as he could rather than have side effects stop him from getting his projects done. He resented the idea of not being able to write due to blisters on his hands and not being able to eat because of blisters in his mouth. They had a solution for that and sent us to the dietician who wanted to give him nourishing drinks full of sugar. We declined the drug Sutent and the sugary drinks. Worried though that he would be totally cut off from the hospital he said ok to trying another medicine with fewer side effects and he started taking Votrient on September 26.

Bad Day
September 15, 2017

*B*ad day!
  Could not eat.
Tired.

Dichotomy

September 20, 2017

*H*ere are two different poems written one day apart. I wanted to post these to show the up and down nature of this whole thing. It's strange how emotions run the gamut from hope to despair and back again. Good days, bad days…one day at a time…that's really all any of us have. I've found that I may venture into the dark places but somehow, and I believe it is because of all the love, thoughts and prayers coming my way, with all your help I find my way back to the light. I am so grateful and humbled by the kindnesses and love I have been shown by so many people. I feel blessed beyond anything I deserve.

"Here's your invitation, start the celebration, this is life!" That was written by a relatively unknown songwriter, but somehow I think he finally got it right. (From Andreas Aleman's album This Is Life, lyrics Brian Hobbs)

TRUE HAPPINESS

A dog in your lap
The memory captured in an old photograph

A call from a friend, a reminder of what has been
The music of Bach, the music of Jarreau
An old blanket, a heater
Being surrounded by things you love and know
The realization that you've lived a good life
That you've been blessed with a caring, devoted wife
Knowing despite the road being dark and long
There are loved ones and friends cheering you on
That if you focus on today
Tomorrow's not so scary
That the load you've been given
Is never more than you can carry
It's knowing that though you never found greatness
You found your place in line
That there are still outbreaks of kindness
And the world offers up treasures
That we still have yet to find

DARKNESS AND LIGHT

You face the darkness and it envelops you to your depths
And you have to fumble and fall, grasping for something, anything to
    hold onto
And you might pray, you might curse, you might long for the peace of
    the abyss
But slowly the eclipse of your soul subsides and the hope still held
    inside you
Tentatively unveils itself in a steady morning rain that washes away
    the stain of night
And the clouds break and the sun finds its feet
And you see God through the diaphanous mist; waving at you
And you can move again, content in the realization that the darkness
    is bound to light
As death is bound to life, that you are momentary and eternal

That you are everything and nothing
That you must embrace your darkness so it can lead you to the light

I Have One Problem

September 21, 2017

I have managed to whittle down all my life's problems to one. It didn't happen by choice, it was imposed on me,
I have kidney cancer metastasized to the liver. All the other things I used to worry about seem pretty insignificant; prestige, money, clothes, pension, work, fame, recognition.

OK, the money thing is always there, but as long as my wife and kids are OK and we can hold onto the house it's good.

I never thought in terms of good days or bad days before, they were just even moving channels carrying me from one place to the next.

Now I see things, sun and shadows, blue skies, rain on a window, the change of seasons. My senses are alive again. Love has gone from abstract to tangible.

Granted, the one problem I have is major, and it's big and ugly and I wrestle with it daily and right now I don't know who has the upper hand, but I know that the Beast feels all the love sent my way and hopefully that is weakening him.

Wishful thinking, Pollyanna dreamer? Maybe, but today is a good day. I'm going to take a walk, and I'm alive to fight another day......and yeah, I still only have one problem.

Started on Drugs

September 26, 2017

September 26—Started taking the drug Votrient.
September 28—Slight burning sensations in hands, itching.
Numbness in toes, drier mouth, more urination at nights.
September 30—Extreme fatigue, irritability.
October 2—Stopped taking it.

Fia's Reflections

Brian's oncologist wanted to start him up on Sutent which is a
medication that can slow down kidney cancer but not cure it. After
much research Brian decided that quality of life was worth so much
more than a bit of extra time and having to deal with severe side effects.
After declining treatment he was offered another medication which
according to the doctor had fewer side effects and he would also only
take half the recommended dose. After thinking about it he decided to
try it and see, but would stop if the side effects were too bad.

After only a day or two Brian turned into a zombie that just sat on
the sofa and did not interact. He became the human vegetable he always

said he did not want to become. After six days on Votrient he stopped taking it and it took a while for him to get back to "normal". In these six short days it affected his thyroid so he had to increase his dose of hormones. It was scary to see the change in him and I was wondering what would have happened if he had taken the full dose.

Kindness and Divine Sparks

September 28, 2017

I'm getting a 3-hour blood transfusion so I have plenty of time to write more random thoughts. Hope you enjoy.

Kindness seems to be an increasingly rare commodity in the world today, but I have been blessed with an abundance of it. Friends and relatives call, send cards, messages, flowers, gifts and food. They give their time unselfishly to stop by and visit, they help with practicalities like groceries and other errands. It's all overwhelming, extremely humbling and wonderful. These people, these divine sparks, send me love and strength by keeping me in their thoughts and prayers. I'm convinced they are a big part of the healing process and I become more thankful every day for having such loving souls in my life. It's hard to stay completely away from my dark places and thoughts, and no matter how hard I try, I sometimes fail miserably and find myself there. But all these divine sparks seem to join forces and lift me out.

Yesterday I got my first good news in a very long time; my liver values improved from 6.9 to 4.4, which is nothing short of a miracle. (The test was taken before I started Votrient). I know this depends on the proactive approach my wife is taking with my home treatment; diet, hyperthermia treatment, hemp oil, and her keeping me grounded. Adjectives to describe her are hard to come by so I have to resort to words like amazing, dedicated and unselfish. She plays a big role, but I cannot forget all my divine sparks; family, friends, colleagues, people in churches who don't even know me, who keep me in their thoughts and prayers. They play an equally important role.

My view of God, the universe, the greater power, whatever you want to call it, has changed. I now see God through kindness, so for me, God is everywhere. I've learned once again that there are many people I belong to.

I still don't know how my story will end, but deep inside I'm positive. All I can do is follow my road and see where it leads. All I can do is buckle up and do my best to squeeze the most life possible out of the time I've been allotted and leave that last page unwritten.

Life is strange. It brings us so many lessons, joys and sorrows, but if we're lucky we find people and things along the way that make the lessons, joys and sorrows worthwhile. Right now I'm one of the luckiest men alive.

Thanks for reading! I love to hear your comments, and thanks for your support and love. It means the world to me.

Fia's Reflections

Since the first day of his diagnosis, Brian opened up to all the help I could offer him. Before he had been stubborn about everything when it came to a healthy diet, exercising and nutrition. After July 17 he was a changed man. We started immediately to change his diet by cutting out sugar, gluten and dairy products. He had no problem doing that at all and went all in and read up on how certain foods affect the body. The only thing he had a problem with were the green juices and he only drank a few with great reluctance now and again. Instead he started taking extra nutrition and a benefit of doing so was that his heart problems went away. After I got him to take Q10 the arrhythmia he had had for years suddenly went away. His heartbeat became regular and the heart operation he had been waiting for during 2017 became unnecessary. He also stopped having sleep apnea due to weight loss.

New Music Coming

September 29, 2017

I just wanted to let everyone know that new music is on the way! The first project out will be a follow-up to my 2003 album, *Impressions of the Outer Banks*, appropriately titled, *Impressions of the Outer Banks II*.

Due to health reasons I'm not really up to recording anything new, but I have looked around and found tracks that have never seen the light of day, including some orchestral sketches I've done over the years. I was unable to afford a real orchestra so the instruments are samples. You see, my pride and fear levels have dropped significantly. I mean what's someone gonna do…give me cancer??? Gallows humor, I know, but I love this music and want to share it with all of you. It will only be released digitally and I'll keep you updated.

I hope to have a little audio teaser to put out within a week or so. Here is the track list just to give you an idea of the direction:

Coquina Beach
Corolla
Sentinels of the Coast

Ghost Ship
Queen Anne's Revenge
Breezin' on a Rainy Day

Once again, thanks for reading my posts. I don't want to wear everyone out with the C word so I just wanted to let you know I'm working hard to try to put together new music for you. As usual, it will be available at www.cdbaby.com, iTunes, Spotify and most other digital streaming sites.

Best, B.

To Be Read at My Memorial Service!
October 1, 2017

I'm a painter with words
I'm a painter of dreams
I look for the eloquence nobody sees
That nobody's seen
I wear the bruises of time
and the scars of love
Still searching for answers to questions
unknown and not giving up
till my story is told

I'm a painter with words
and my palette is life
I paint all the beauty, the wrongs and the rights
in shadows and lights
My canvas the depths of my soul
and my heart's desires
I write of lost innocence

39

the ebb and the flow
And search for the truth
till my story is told

I see into tomorrow
I walk in yesterday
I echo rolling thunder
On the cold and empty page
But most of all
most of all

I'm a painter with words
I'm a painter of dreams
I look for the eloquence nobody sees
That nobody's seen
I wear the bruises of time
and the scars of love
Still searching for answers to questions
unknown and not giving up
till my story is told

Fia's Reflections

Our son Adam read this poem at the memorial service in Stockholm held on April 21, 2018.

Too Tired

October 2, 2017

Too tired!

Fia's Reflections

This is when Brian decided to stop the drug Votrient after six days. He had no strength to do anything and the writing he had enjoyed was now an enormous effort. "Feeling like this I might as well be dead already" he said. He was a shadow of himself and could not do anything so he stopped taking it.

An Explanation and a Thank You.

October 4, 2017

When I was first diagnosed with cancer I was told there was no cure, that the best I could hope for was to slow it down and buy more time until the inevitable. But I had so much support and love from friends and relatives that I began to believe otherwise. The prayers have been overwhelming.

Even so, I felt I had to do certain things, and one of these was to put the logistics of death and dying behind me. So I got my affairs in order and went about talking to people I loved, and in essence, getting the goodbyes out of the way. I wanted nothing left unsaid. Some people have misunderstood this as giving up. It's not. For me, it was a stage where I had to release myself from life so I could focus on living. So I'm sorry if anyone felt I was giving up. If anything, my faith and belief is stronger than ever. We are fighting this thing with everything we've got. Plus, there are all my divine sparks. And I will never underestimate them again. Not giving up!

I received a package today from one of my cousins. It came at exactly the right time. The side effects of my medication kicked in full force this past weekend and I have been so extremely tired I haven't even been able to function. In this package was a prayer cloth (a handkerchief from my mother), a tangible reminder of all the people praying for me, people whom in many cases I don't even know. It was a strong reminder of how loving, unselfish and kind people can be. And when it comes to family I am amazingly blessed. We may not see each other often, but when there is sickness or need they are always there. This package, which also contained an inspirational book, may seem like a small, insignificant gesture, but for me it offered renewed hope and led me out of a series of dark days; just another ordinary miracle. I've been experiencing more and more of those lately.

This is a humbling time in my life, but I also feel elevated. It's good to be reminded, despite all the hatred and senseless killing we see, that there is love and there are still people who care. Thanks Janus!

What's in a Day?

October 5, 2017

I'll admit, I'd never thought about that question until today. If you're reading this then you probably know I have cancer, a kamikaze pilot from hell. Its only goal seems to be to kill you and itself. Well... enough of that.

Back to what's in a day. My day has become more finite. It revolves around much fewer things like food, medicine, exercise and trying to keep my brain and creativity in shape. I have to take small breaks and lay down to rest. I purposely avoid TV during the day. Instead, I listen to music that moves me and try to write.

I guess the biggest change in my day's pre-C and post-C is that I'm forced to face my mortality every morning. It's quite liberating actually. You lose many of your fears. You also think more about living rather than working, about loving rather than co-existing, about being rather than doing. I've become more aware, more thoughtful and thankful. Don't get me wrong, I have not found Nirvana nor have my inner demons given up the ghost. It's a daily battle, and right now, riding on two weeks of improved liver and blood values, I'd say I'm slightly ahead.

A day can be filled with many things. Like life, a day can consist of tears, despair, good times and laughter. I think it's good for all of us to look at our days and take a little inventory. Maybe it's time to throw out the bad stock, or replenish supplies. Maybe we've run low on passion, hope, understanding, curiosity? Those are items we need in stock every day. We need to develop the eloquence of our souls so that we can truly speak.

No one is promised tomorrow so one day at a time is really all we can expect. Savor it, make it special. Share a kindness. Take a little time to look inside yourself and evolve and grow. Easier said than done I know, and I'm certainly not there yet, but I'm trying to live a lifetime in a day and look at a day as a lifetime. That sounds weird but maybe someone will understand what I'm trying to say.

Thanks for listening to yet more of my random thoughts. It's my therapy and if it helps someone going through the same thing then that's an added plus. I love to get your comments so please write! Thanks. B.

Fia's Reflections

I took me by surprise when Brian started to blog about his cancer as we both like our privacy. I guess he decided to make it easy for his family, friends and all the people he had met over the years to be open and let them know instead of speculating. I think anyone who blogs about their illness is brave. I also know how much healing and grief processing it entails for the person writing it as well as for people who read it. Brian's blog made a change in so many people's lives and I am very proud of him for facing his fears and going through with it. As he said in a previous blog, "my pride and fear levels have dropped significantly. I mean what's someone gonna do…give me cancer??"

Most of the time our fears hold us back from doing what we really want to do and our minds are many times excellent at showing a scenario that COULD happen if we dared to try. Our brain tries to protect us which is good when it comes to really dangerous situations. But it can also act like an overprotective mother hen at times when the fear prevents you from taking a new chance, a new job, holding a speech or reaching out to someone in case you would fail or get rejected. What is the worst thing that can happen? A rejection is not going to kill you.

A Cautious Peek into the Future

October 6, 2017

I wrote earlier about the importance of living one day at a time, and now I'm going to talk about something very contradictory: planning for the future.

One of the first and hardest things I did after learning my kidney cancer had spread to my liver was start planning for my death. The will was simple, but the power of attorney, insurance and financial stuff was a jungle. I coped pretty well until I got around to planning my own memorial service. Yes, I did that because I wanted to save my family from one other thing to have to deal with. I completely broke down. But that was also where a change occurred. I gained hope again and put death and dying behind me. I acknowledged it and faced down this giant, ugly fear and it became just a "thing".

After that I could focus on living, on trying to get better and I believe that's when the real healing started. I started to feel the strength and love of all of you I refer to as my divine sparks. I started making plans again. I started thinking about new albums. I forced myself to get up and walk. I refused to get in my bed during the day.

I am still focused on my day to day living but I also dare to take a cautious peek into the future. By doing that I found my hope again. I found I could still believe in miracles. But I also realized that miracles demand hard work and commitment.

And I sincerely hope you don't think that I'm telling you "I've got all this figured out". I don't. I just want to share my thoughts and experiences in the desire that they just might help someone going through the same thing.

I'm learning, I'm struggling and I'm stumbling my way through this. I need all the help I can get so please keep the prayers and good thoughts coming. They mean more to me than any of you know.

Thanks for all the comments. I'm sorry I can't respond to each and every one, but I read them all and they always lighten my day. Thank you from the bottom of my heart!

B.

Fia's Reflections

Facing your fears head-on instead of dodging them can be daunting at first, but once you have started you can scale it down and move through them one step at time. Brian did just that when he started planning his memorial services, one for his family and friends in Elizabeth City in North Carolina, and the other one to be held in Stockholm. He showed it to me and even if it was tough to read it I was happy he took the time to write it down so it would turn out the way he wanted it to be and that I did not have make those decisions.

It was a big load that had been taken off his shoulders and there were more things we looked into, in case of his death. We wanted to take care of as much as possible to make it easier for us who would be left behind. There were many tears but also a sense of taking control over a situation that no one really knew how or when it would end.

Rediscovery

October 9, 2017

What a wonderful word. For me, it means realizing and appreciating things I never gave a second thought to before; having an appetite, sleeping and other bodily functions. I have also rediscovered the importance of friendships and relationships. I also take time to think, to be aware. Except for major events I stay away from the filler and bulls*** from both sides of the political spectrum. That alone has given me a great deal of peace of mind. I've rediscovered that worry is a waste. I'm learning that finding a purpose is the greatest gift.

Quite simply, I'm rediscovering myself, complete with all the flaws and self-inflicted wounds. And I'm healing, not only in my body but in my soul. I'm no longer crippled by doubts and fears. Acceptance is a big part of my daily life. Abandoned dreams have been rediscovered. I've fallen in love with words again and they take me deep inside myself so I can look out and see all the things I'd forgotten.

Rediscovery, maybe it's part of the evolution of life. Maybe it's the thing that renews us or let's us see once again through the soul of a child.

So take the time today to rediscover yourself. You might be surprised at what you find.

Thanks again for reading and I love to get your comments!

Love, B.

Fia's Reflections

I was happy to see Brian come to life again after the short but totally devastating medication he took during six days. He was grateful that he could write again and he wanted to get more projects done in the time he had left, however long that would be. He also went on a deep discovery inside himself and I cannot begin to tell what a different man it was that came out. Brian had always been the sweetest man but now a whole new curious side appeared and he began to take an interest in things he had not been into before. His transformation into a deeply spiritual being accelerated in a short time and he achieved a deep understanding that often takes a lifetime to reach.

The Taste of Fruit Stripe Gum

October 11, 2017

*Y*ou all have been kind enough to read my "random thoughts" and I've gotten some really nice comments about my writing. So, I thought I would try something new. Most people don't know that in addition to music and lyrics I also write poetry and prose. Here is a story I wrote a number of years ago. So far it's the first and only story of mine that has been published in a literary magazine. (The Sierra Nevada Review, Volume 20—2009). I hope you'll take the time to read it and please feel free to tell me whether or not you'd like more things like this.

THE TASTE OF FRUIT STRIPE GUM
By Brian Hobbs

He'd always hated that smell; the smell of old people, the stuffy, musty smell of antiseptic cleaners, decay and old sweat. It had always made him feel claustrophobic. He remembered the interminable sessions his grandmother had made him endure by taking him to visit old aunts and uncles and other assorted relatives that he had no interest in knowing and who talked about people he'd never heard

51

of and events he knew nothing about. It seemed old people were deathly afraid of drafts and there was never any air in these places. In the summer the air was stale and the windows covered to keep out the heat. In winter, the air was stale and the windows covered to keep in the heat.

He'd gotten the same instructions every time; sit still, say sir and ma'am, and never touch anything. She'd also instructed him to always accept money from them if they offered. This last instruction was added after he had been offered a quarter by some ancient relative and had declined to accept by saying, "no thank you, I have my own money".

Most of the houses they visited were shingled and made of wood except for a couple of older relatives who lived in the new projects. The interiors usually consisted of a settee and one or two straight-back chairs, an easy chair and a coffee table. The wallpaper was usually some kind of dark, overdone floral pattern. Sometimes a radio show was playing low in the background; Christian music where a man sang, "In times like these, we need a Savior" and "Softly and tenderly Jesus is calling." Other times it was just the sound of a clock ticking and the squeak of an old rocker.

He liked visiting one old aunt because she had a glass cabinet with figurines. There was a white carriage drawn by four, ceramic white horses, complete with a driver and coachman, also in white, but with painted faces and uniforms trimmed in gold. There was a pair of dogs with golden ears and noses with black eyes. She also had two glass kittens, one blue and one pink, that he was allowed to play with. The aunt's name might have been Maggie. Aunt Maggie, if that was her name, was his favorite. Sometimes she would even crawl down on the floor and play with him. All the others just sat there in the stifling heat of summer with the drapes pulled and one pathetic electric fan that merely moved the dead, sickly air from one side of the room to the other. In winter it was worse; the hot, heavy air didn't move at all.

The majority of the old people just sat in their chairs and stared out at him. This always scared him because he felt that they weren't looking at him but looking through him. The old women, when they did speak, spoke in raspy, slurred voices. To him it sounded like every breath was a struggle. When they weren't talking they kept moving their fat tongues around in their mouths like they were trying to create a little moisture so they would be able to speak. Their eyes seemed to have a shiny, bluish film over them. Even in all the heat, the men wore black jackets and ties and the women wore dark, long-sleeved dresses. The women's hair was gray, pulled back tight from their faces in a severe bun that was done up with all types of nets and pins and clips and their skin was pallid like the wax, white candles on the birthday cake his grandmother had made him. Some of the people had strange faces that didn't move, and when they spoke only one side of their lips moved. He hated visiting these people because they reminded him of the scary clowns at the amusement park or the clowns who rode in the trucks for the potato festival or Christmas parade. He hated the fact that sometimes they called him by other names and talked to him about things he'd never done and people he never knew.

He had been scared to death on one visit to someone his grandmother referred to as Uncle Ivey. This man had one whole side of his face missing. It looked like his head had just caved in. When the boy saw him he'd started crying and run back to the car but his grandmother came out and got him. She explained, "Son, Uncle Ivey was eat up with the cancer and he's lucky to be alive. They had to cut away half his face but the doctors say Uncle Ivey's all right now. Through the grace of the Lord and the power of prayer they took all the cancer and he's going to live."

The boy calmed down but still wondered what cancer was. By that time, Uncle Ivey had come out to the car and was offering him a pack of Beech Nut Fruit Stripe gum. That had helped. He really liked the lime. He went with his grandmother inside and visited and tried not to look at Uncle Ivey. As a reward, on the way home his grandmother stopped at the Sundry Shop and bought him a fountain coke.

The worst visit was always to his grandmother's half-sister. Her name was Viola. Her husband had left her and run off with "that woman" that worked at the dry-cleaners. Aunt Viola and her ex-husband had had a son, Herbert Ray, who was just a few years older than the boy. Herbert Ray was sick. He was always in pajamas and the house was always dark and even though Aunt Viola was younger than the boy's grandmother, her house smelled like an "old people" house. Herbert Ray was pale with dark eyes and greasy hair. The boy was horribly afraid of him, thought he was one of the demons the preachers talked about in church. Everywhere Herbert Ray went in the house he had to carry a bucket in case he vomited. Eventually, Herbert Ray died. Aunt Viola met a preacher, got married again and moved to Tennessee. His grandmother had taken him to visit Aunt Viola right before she moved away with the preacher, and even with Herbert Ray being dead, Aunt Viola seemed a lot happier and it was the first time the boy ever remembered seeing her smile.

He missed his grandmother. She'd died from an aneurysm when he was 15. She never really got old enough to smell or look like all the relatives she and he used to visit. She was in the kitchen fixing pickles one day and just keeled over dead. He'd cried when he saw her in the casket and thought his heart would break when they clamped shut the lid to the coffin and he knew he would never see her again.

God, how he wished he could have gone like that. Instead, he'd been brought to this place. He couldn't remember his name, or who his children were, but he remembered the smell; antiseptic cleaners, decay and old sweat. He didn't know the name of the old uncle he saw in the mirror and sat with all day. He wore a stained striped tie and an old black suit jacket and stared back through rheumy eyes from inside his pale skin.

He missed his grandmother. She was about the only person he still remembered. He always wore an old pair of sunglasses because his eyes were so sensitive to the light. At least that's what he told people. Actually the sunglasses served as a kind of wall to insulate him from all these people. He didn't want them near him; he still hated their smell.

After he'd eaten the food he could no longer taste, he sat in his chair until the lights went out at 7:00. He was put into his bed but he didn't sleep. He stared into the dark and tried to remember the taste of Fruit Stripe gum.

A Poem

October 11, 2017

We can't see the tide that moves beneath the wave
We can't see the wind that drives clouds

Got an Idea

October 12, 2017

*g*ot an idea for doing Independent* as a concert version in EC. (Elizabeth City, North Carolina).

1.5 hours of music
  30 minutes of exposition
  2.15 max show
  15 minutes intermission
  Need 5000 dollars to finish recording score
  3 woodwinds
  1 violin
  2 brass
  drums

The Independent Man, a musical Brian wrote about the newspaperman W.O Saunders in Elizabeth City. He finally released the music on November 30, 2017 on CD Baby and Spotify.

His dream was that it would be set up in his hometown as a musical but he had no luck in getting interest and money. On this day he came up with the idea about a concert version but unfortunately he was not able to go further with the idea.

Ordinary Miracles

October 13, 2017

*W*ell, for the fourth week in a row my liver values improved. In four weeks things have gone from 6.9 to 4.4 to 3.5 to 3.0. A half percentage point may seem insignificant, but for me, with what I'm going through, it's enough to plan a celebration around. The top of the value range for normal people is around 1.9.

For me, this is nothing short of a miracle since in late August I was basically given a death sentence. I am taking a proactive approach with diet, what exercise I can do, as well as other things. I know that is helping, but I also know that all the prayers and love being sent my way are playing a major role. So I'd like to give my heartfelt thanks to everyone who is praying for me, for all the prayer lists I'm on and for all the support and love I get from friends and family. I know I still have a long way to go (it's actually only been a little over two months since the operation). But I am extremely positive and my faith and belief is stronger than ever. Sincere thanks for all the flowers, visits, gifts, food, calls and messages. This whole journey has been miraculous to say the least. It's changed me as a person (for the better).

I still have my good days and bad days, but in general, the good outweighs the bad. I am so thoughtful and thankful that things seem to be moving in the right direction. By the way, today is setting up to be a good day. I could eat breakfast, I feel pretty good, some wonderful former students of mine are coming for a visit, and I'm getting ready to take my walk. I can listen to music, plan my new album and most importantly, I'm living.

Thanks for everything. I do love to read your comments so please write! Have a great weekend and let someone know you love them. It will do both of you a lot of good. Listen to music, it's a great healer. Make sure you are living not just existing.

Fia's Reflections

To be given hope, support and love are three good ingredients for creating miracles.

Without hope—what is the use of trying?

Without support—you don't get far.

Without love—life is less colorful.

Brian thrived on hearing from people that were reading his blog as it was his way of having contact with the outside world. He would only see a few visitors as he wanted to stay away from being exposed to infections and colds. He felt deeply surrounded by love and the more he expressed it, the more it came back. It was a beautiful experience.

A Thought

October 14, 2017

This thought came to mind today:

I've discovered the importance of... (Fill in the blank with your own words).

For me the list would be long.

Friends and Family: This One's for You

October 16, 2017

I've seen and read about so many people who shut themselves away after getting a serious disease. Of course, sometimes it's necessary because you're physically unable to see people. I'm thankful that except for certain times I've not had to do that and I think it's helped the healing process.

Seeing and talking to friends is energizing, it makes me happy. I may be physically tired after the visit or call but I get so much internal and emotional strength. Sharing a laugh with friends is the best medicine I know. I am greatly humbled that people take the time to stop by or talk to me on the phone, that they send me love and strength in their comments to this blog and Facebook, that they pray for me and send cards and flowers. I can't overexaggerate what it means to me. The personal connection is a huge thing and that is why I'm so grateful for friends and family.

That's why I wanted to devote today to all of you. You are such a big part of my life, and that includes all the new friends I haven't met yet, people I've come into contact with through this blog. So I've attached an audio file that I hope you will listen to that I recorded a couple of years ago. It's called "MIRACLES", and that's what all of you are; my divine sparks. I hope you enjoy it and that it brings you just a small touch of the comfort and light all of you have brought to me. Humble thanks and much love!

Brian

Fia's note: the song Miracles was never released officially

Too Many "Metoos"

October 17, 2017

*D*eeply saddened and troubled by how many "me too" statuses I have seen over the last few days. I cannot comprehend the pain and suffering all this must have caused, especially since it happened for many of the victims when they were quite young. There is never any age when it is right but to violate a child is truly abhorrent.

I am impressed by women's bravery and solidarity. I believe a change will come, the real change has to come from us men. Until we face the problem and our own attitudes no lasting change can occur. Guys, we own this, we have propagated it. Only we can fix it. I don't have the solution but I know it starts with awareness. Laws have to change. Equality and respect have to be embraced.

I am certainly ready for another approach. Making sexual harassment and assault a thing of the past doesn't take a miracle, all it requires is a conscious effort to make a change.

Five Fears

October 18, 2017

1. That I will never feel good again.
2. That I will waste away to a corpse.
3. That I'll never be able to write again.
4. That I will not have the energy to do my work.
5. That I will lose my faith (crossed out).

Fears

October 19, 2017

Written Tuesday, October 17

Tuesdays are always days of anguish for me. That's when I get my weekly blood tests. I hope the values keep improving but I know it's not always a straight path, so like the weather in Stockholm, my mood is dark.

I'm more tired than usual and have been feeling nauseous, it's like a veil has been put over my spirit. I realize I have to do the only thing I can do, just breathe. The breathing helps and I start thinking about my happy places. But today they are all blurred and seem to fade away. And then the tears start. I go in to talk to my wife, who is not only my wife but my therapist and psychologist. She asks me to write down my five biggest fears, which I do. She then proceeds to show me one by one how all these fears are locked up in the future; that I more than likely will not die today, that today I can still function, that I can still write, that I still have my faith (it's just slightly weakened), that maybe the reason I don't feel as good as I would like is…SURPRISE…I have cancer. She tells me the fears are driven by imagination. She also tells me that if I start living in the world of "what might happen" that I will miss all the good things in this life. She does this with love and a smile but also with a look that says "you better remember all this because today is where you are, it's where we all are until our time comes".

She's a wise woman. Now the fears are like the majority of the cancer cells we all carry: they're there but dormant and harmless. It's when we let them take over that they grow and start to eat us up.

I have two words I'd like to add to my profile; cancer-free and fearless. I am grateful to my wife for making me feel like both are a possibility. Please continue to keep us in your thoughts and prayers.

Love, B.

Fia's Reflections

The way to inner peace is not a straight line. During a day you can have feelings ranging from happiness, worry and fear and it can go round in circles many times. The first step in being able to deal with the tougher and unwanted emotions is to acknowledge them as having a right to show up. The next thing is to examine them and see them for what they are, a response to thoughts you have. We have between 25 000 to 50 000 thoughts in a day and they all affect how we feel.

A good way to take a look at what is going on with you is to write down the fears you have and what thoughts come up as negative mantras in your head. Ask yourself if your thoughts/beliefs are true, if they help you feel the way you want to feel, if they help you reach your short and long term goals.

By breaking down every fear and sentence you have written, it takes the edge off and you are able to deal with them differently. Some can be discarded entirely while others you learn to cope with. I do recommend you talk to a therapist if you feel this is hard to do on your own. The reason you can feel stuck is because you are in the middle of it, and it takes someone from the outside to help you look at it from another angle or come to acceptance when that is needed.

I helped Brian with his list and gave him skills to cope and get rid of a few, while others he learned to live with and look at differently.

Something We All Can Do...
Live This Life!

October 22, 2017

Some days you just want the struggle and routine to end. You don't want to eat. You don't want to exercise. You don't want to live. But as this wise woman keeps telling me, you have to look at what you can do, like me writing this piece. And I'll admit it, when she tells me that stuff it pisses me off because I'm all ready to wallow in self-pity and desperation and she ruins it for me. I'm lying there ready to waste away and suddenly I'm getting dressed to take my walk. I'm all ready to curse God and the universe for imposing this disease on me and instead I find myself thankful I can move.

This "she" is my wife and I'm blessed to have her.

As I wrote the other day and will post later, there will be dark days, but as tired, weak and frustrated as I get there are always things to be thankful for, always something I can do.

A Look into the Dark Days

October 23, 2017

I try to be as honest as I can here, so I wanted to show that there are dark sides to this journey. This is a poem I wrote in the early days. I don't visit here so often anymore. I've been blessed with miracles, love and hope, but this is how you feel when the doctors say things like, "there is no cure, the best you can hope for is that we can slow things down" and "I'm sorry if I sound harsh, but you'll never feel normal again". I don't blame them, they're doing their jobs, but they obviously did not take into account all the divine sparks in my life. Thank you all once again! But here's a look into the dark side.

CANCER

The world crumbles and you are falling
You're surrounded by debris
Your limbs are lifeless strings
Hanging from your body
Your mind is clear and you see a manic
slide show of scenes from your life

as you continue to fall
You keep waiting for a lifeline
and sleep is the only freedom you find
You remember the bible study from your
childhood about Gilead
You only remember the question
"Is there balm in Gilead?"
You don't know where Gilead is but if
there is balm there you want to go
You've lost more weight than you want to mention,
but feel heavier than you've ever felt
The days are endless and there's nothing you
can do except watch your descent
You look down but there is no bottom
so you reconcile yourself to the falling
Over and over with the broken remnants
of yourself strewn about you

Happy Tears

October 25, 2017

*T*oday I woke up in tears, not out of despair but because I was so overwhelmingly happy. I am still amazed at the outpouring of love and generosity, that people can be so kind and compassionate. In the midst of the darkest period of my life I have been given so much. I am closer to friends, family and God. I see my purpose clearly. I think doing this little tango with death has made me more alive. Like a song I wrote for a character in my musical…"and one day soon I'll pay the fare like the visionaries who searched for truth, teachers, poets, kings and dukes. I may not get it right, but I'm here to live this life".

See what you can do today, and most importantly…live your life.

Thanks for following my journey and for all your kind and supportive comments.

Love, B.

The Most Lonesome Sound—
A Story From A Few Years Back

October 26, 2017

The most lonesome sound has to be a train whistle…and not just any train whistle…but a southern train whistle.

The last time I heard one was this June in Nashville, Tennessee. If you've never heard it, it's the most heartbreaking sound on earth, filled with the smell of rain on magnolias, summer sweat and the feverish chill of a night breeze in high summer. I heard it and it transported me back home, a home of crickets and bullfrogs, the sound of a car rattling down a dirt road with the fading wail of music from a radio, a home of a million stars thrown on a black sky and the smell of summer rain on hot asphalt, a home with an alabaster moon rising from behind the pines.

When I was young we used to live off Church Street Extended and the railroad tracks ran less than half a mile in front of our house. As a child, before we had air-conditioning, I remember lying in bed on summer nights, the sheets damp and twisted, windows open and the sound of evening pouring in; the gentle swish of the branches of a weeping willow, the night birds and distant howling of a dog. And on those late nights when I laid in my bed with my eyes shut tight trying to see God, sometimes I would hear the moan of the whistle as the train reached the crossing. It was haunting and beautiful, a sound that moved me but also a sound I did not yet understand.

My father told me once of the way the train whistles sounded when he was young, when the trains came through town carrying the bodies of soldiers who had been killed in the war to their final resting place. He said the engineers on those trains had a way of making that whistle cry, and somehow that cry carried all the anguish and pain of those dead boys' lost dreams, the unimaginable sorrow of never loving a woman, never holding a child, never seeing home again. My father told me he would never forget that sound.

Somehow I think those whistles still echo throughout the south, moaning and crying for the memory of the Native Americans who once lived on this land, who are now forgotten and only live on in place names like Pasquotank, Currituck, Perquimans, Hatteras and Chowan, for the black men and women, enslaved and used, worn out and tossed away by misguided, arrogant, cruel and selfish men of another color, for the men, women and children who suffered and worked in the cotton mills, for the poor farmers toiling on the land, for the young soldiers who fought for a lost cause, caught up in the grandeur of the uncompromising rantings of old men that split a country in half, for the lovers whose stars never collided, for all the pain and hurt that's just as much a part of this land as the grass, azaleas, cypress and pine trees and lazy rivers.

That lonesome whistle still echoes the sorrows and joys of the proud people who came from this land and returned to it; ashes to ashes, dust to dust.

A southern train whistle…it has to be the most lonesome sound I've ever heard.

A Dark Day!

October 27, 2017

A dark day!

Fia's Reflections

We visited the oncologist and she more or less gave Brian the boot. It is not what you say, it is how you say it! Total devastation for the next three days.

During the seven months Brian lived with his diagnosis he experienced many ups and downs. I realized early on that if he was going to make it at all I needed to be there to be his wife, his coach, his therapist and listening friend. I was not able to keep up with my work so I decided to spend the time with Brian as I did not know how much longer he had left to live.

The decision was easy, the economic reality harsh. Had it not been for family and friends we would not have survived and we solved problems one day at a time. One friend came by frequently with home-cooked food to make it easy for me to focus on caring for Brian and he kept it up for months. Others gave money, groceries and also sent me off to a spa for half a day. That came at a particularly rough time just after we had had a tough meeting with his oncologist who did not see any point in Brian getting any more checkups. He was devastated and close to giving up. It took three rough days before both of us could shake off her words and start living life the best we could.

Although we did not know how things were going to turn out when we started, we still felt fortunate for having friends and family who cared. To open up and ask for help is one of the hardest things to do but the gifts were all given with so much love and respect for our situation that we gladly accepted it.

I'll Keep on Livin'

October 29, 2017

When I started writing this blog I promised myself I would always be honest. I got bad news on Friday. My disease is progressing rapidly and I am being transferred to palliative care. The change over the last few days has been dramatic. It's amazing to see your body fail you. Taking food has turned into a major struggle. The slightest thing will bring on nausea; an undercooked vegetable, the smell of a certain spice, if the texture is wrong.

Writing this used to be a joy, now every line tires me out. This is a hateful and relentless disease. I asked the doctor on Friday how the time frame was looking for this thing: her answer was "anything from a matter of months to a year". I wanted to know but it still shakes you to your core when they put a number on it.

Fia's Reflections

On October 27 we went to see the oncologist for the second time and also the last. The news was bad and it was heartbreaking to see Brian's mood change and how it affected his whole quality of life. It was like turning a corner because immediately he felt his body failing him in every single way as described by him above. We had long talks on how nocebo (when you expect the worst to happen) plays a big role in these circumstances and he was definitely under the spell for a solid three days. We talked about the fact that he will die but that it was not going to happen today.

The same day we came home from that fatal meeting with the oncologist, a friend who is an acupuncturist came over and helped us get through the day by giving us both some bodywork. Because of Brian's total drop in mood I was shocked to see how quickly his body started failing him. It was instantaneous. Everything from his posture to not being able to eat, feeling nauseous etc. This was very hard for me to watch and during the weekend my mood and energy also failed.

That Sunday my sister came to visit and we went to a spa as I had gotten a gift certificate from some friends. It saved me! For the first time I could get away and think about me and take care of myself. I scrubbed, I sweated, and I steamed and finally went swimming. After a few hours I felt cleansed and I had a chance to talk about mine and Brian's situation and what to expect next. When I got back home my energy was increased and I could be a good support again. I promised myself to make this a habit but in retrospect that did not happen due to a lack of money and time.

The following day, on October 30, I started looking around for palliative care and on November 8 we had the first home visit from the palliative care team.

There is a dilemma for caregivers as it is difficult to care for someone and at the same time care for yourself. I don't have an easy answer to this. In theory, yes, ask for help, get someone to pick up groceries or have them delivered, pamper yourself with massage or any other treatment, take long walks, talk to a friend or a professional, get your whole family involved etc.

In practice the answer is whatever gets you through the day and the next and don't be hard on yourself. You are coping the best way you can.

Not My Day to Die

October 30, 2017

I feel better today and as I woke up I was reminded of the last line in my favorite authors' (William Styron) novel, Sophie's Choice: "This was not judgement day—only morning. Morning: excellent and fair". Not my day to die.

I'll Keep on Livin' Lyrics
October 31, 2017

*T*his song pretty much sums up how I feel right now so I'll let it do its work.

I'LL KEEP ON LIVIN'

I'm walking on a high wire looking everywhere but down
Can't fly away and I don't wanna hit the ground
So I just gotta get across this damn thing
Find a way to the other side
Gotta keep on moving forward cause ain't no place left to hide
I'm sitting on a storm cloud
And I'm bruised black and blue
Gotta heal this broken heart
Maybe change my point of view
So reach out for another star
Get acquainted with the night
Try to reconcile the fact that
I might never get it right

I'll keep on living
Sometimes I'm swimming underwater

I try to hold my breath
Looking for the answer
But I ain't found nothing yet
But one day I'll cross that Jordan
And I'll see the Promised Land
Even though I may not get there
I gotta take the chance
I'll keep on living

Music and lyrics Brian Hobbs

Time Seems to Melt

October 31, 2017

Time seems to melt
shredding small layers
as I move through the passages
toward what is to be

Profound Experience

November 9, 2017

I had a profound experience last night. My American family came to visit yesterday so it was pretty emotional. They brought cards and letters from people in the US. Anyway, in the dead of night I woke up and could not sleep and I started just being thankful for everything and suddenly I felt all this love wash over me and then came this feeling of complete peace and healing. It was wonderful and I knew that in whatever direction this thing takes it's all good.

I have had bad days where the tiredness took over but mentally and spiritually I am strong. I have gained a lot of strength from my family and my party, maybe not in body, but in spirit. I got a new writing desk today that allows me to write comfortably, so I hope there will be more entries.

I still need your prayers. Please keep the divine sparks burning.

Love, B

Fia's Reflections

On November 8 we got the first visit from the palliative cancer care team that makes house calls. We met the doctor and a nurse who would be our main contact and they set up a schedule that a nurse would come by every Thursday to make sure Brian had everything he needed and they would also be able to take his blood tests so he would not have to leave the house for that.

The day after, Brian's parents, sister and niece came to visit from the States and I was not sure how his parents would react to seeing Brian. It was an emotional meeting and I think they were shocked to see him looking so marred by the disease.

It was tears of joy and sadness. His parents managed to make the trip although they are in their early eighties and we all knew that this was going to be the last time they saw each other. They wanted to make this Thanksgiving something special and planned for a big dinner on November 11 that turned out to be everything we hoped for and more. Brian will write about it in the next chapter.

One of the Best Days of My Life
November 12, 2017

*M*embers of my family (my mother, father, sister and niece) are here visiting and yesterday we had an early Thanksgiving together with a few close friends. We had a lot of laughs, a few tears and great food. There was so much warmth and love in that room. But the big surprise was when many of my musician friends showed up and performed. I was literally moved to tears.

I am still amazed at the outpouring of love from everyone. It truly has healing power. They sang my songs and I cried. I was touched beyond description.

Kindness and love…two of the most wonderful things on earth!

Major thanks to Andreas Aleman for arranging the whole thing, and to Wojtek Goral, Teresa Perrelli, Mia Löfgren, Peter Getz, Tom Levin, Johan Becker and Charlotte Berg and other friends for making my day…one of the best days of my life! I love you all. And thanks to my family for making the effort to come visit and for giving me that day. You all are loved more than you know.

And to my immediate family, I love you more than I can express. Love you Fia, Adam and Jeremy!

Fia's Reflections

I was a bit apprehensive when Andreas approached me about the plan of surprising Brian by inviting friends to play and sing for him as his health was quite fragile and I never knew from day to day if he would be able to even attend the planned Thanksgiving dinner. I decided to say yes and get Brian in the best possible shape I could.

On that day he was very tired but I managed to get him out and go to the place we had rented close by. It was the immediate family and some close friends who were invited for the dinner. After we were done the singers and musicians showed up. Brian had no idea they were coming and to see his face and how overwhelmed he was by the outpouring of love and music was amazing. He had earlier during the dinner been thanking everyone and told all of us what we meant to him. It was his way of saying goodbye and we all sat with tears in our eyes. It was both a painful and beautiful moment with lots of feelings to handle.

His family stayed for a week and left on November 15 and from then on Brian's health went quickly downhill.

Messages

November 20, 2017

*T*oday, I received messages from three friends that came when I most needed them. Thanks to Titti Blom for her lovely song, Jonas Gideon for his kind words and Monica Silverstrand for her lovely video. I love all of you. Thanks! Brian

The First Death

November 23, 2017

Fia's Reflections

Today is Thanksgiving in the States and it is also the birthday of Brian's father who turns 82. Brian gave up today mentally and physically, and wanted us all to be there to say goodbye. While one of my sons sat by his bed and having what Brian thought would be his last conversation, I was on the phone trying to get our other son to come home but he could not make it until the day after.

I sat with Brian and we said our goodbyes, I told him he would have to wait until tomorrow to see his other son. Even though I knew this day was coming and had been preparing myself the best I could, it still shook me hard and I was in tears most of the day. It was the first of five tough close to death experiences that we had in front of us. The others would come in January.

No matter how much you prepare yourself it will still be hard when the time comes. With Brian we had several close to death scares and each time it got a little bit easier to handle as we knew that the relief of death was welcomed by Brian. It is very important to reach acceptance and that goes for the person being sick as well as for the family. It makes the passing easier for all and a chance to make it serene and peaceful.

Once our other son got home the next day and Brian was able to have a final talk to him, Brian's anguish seemed to slowly diminish. He was laying in bed that whole weekend not able to get up or eat anything. The boys and I did the best we could to take care of him but also to keep our spirits up. We sat in the same room and played a game one night and laughed and talked. Brian told us later on that hearing us gave him a spark to fight and not give up. Brian writes about his change in his blog entry from December 9.

Three days after he thought he would die, he got up to eat and wanted to sit down and go through his music files. On November 28 his album Healing Purpose came out on Spotify and the following days I helped him with more practical things in regards to his music.

Another songwriter, Erica Iljero Winberg, sent a beautiful version of a song that she and Brian had written years earlier. She recorded it acapella and sent it to Brian on this Sunday. We both cried and said at the same time that this should absolutely be played at the funeral and memorial, and it was. The song is called "Something Along the Way" and it still affects me deeply.

Recovering from My Healing
December 2, 2017

*T*he myriad of emotions I feel sometimes leave me breathless
　　I hear the conversations and laughter from my family
Am moved by the simple joys of a meal together
Am amazed that I am still alive, still fighting
I have decided I am recovering from my healing
Call me a fool but I believe in miracles
I believe in God and I believe in my purpose
I have a mantra that I have spoken and continue to speak more than
I can remember:

"I have a purpose, God gave me this purpose, I know my purpose,
My purpose is to help other people find their own purpose."

It's simple but it has become clear to me…
Recovering from my healing, perhaps a strange way of looking
at things,

But right now I feel like living out my purpose is my sole (or soul) purpose

Continue to pray for me and send me strength. I need all my divine sparks pulling for me. Thanks for the love!

Brian

An Early Christmas Gift to All My Divine Sparks

December 3, 2017

*H*ere is a version of me doing *Silent Night* featuring my talented and great friend, Wojtek Goral on sax. Hope you enjoy. He's amazing and I love him like a brother! Thanks Wojtek! I owe you a bottle of you know what.

SILENT NIGHT featuring Wojtek Goral can be found on Spotify under Brian's name.

Fia's Reflections

Since November 23 when Brian thought he would not survive another day, he managed to turn his life around and see what he still was able to do and realized he was not ready to give up just yet. He asked me and the boys for permission to die and we gave it to him with our hearts. He was ready and we accepted it. Still there was something that brought him back. His purpose in life was getting stronger and he kept repeating it for himself as a mantra:

I have a purpose, God gave me this purpose, I know my purpose,
My purpose is to help other people find their own purpose.

On this day during his afternoon healing hour in my healing room, he sprung a total surprise on me. Laying there on the bench he asked me to marry him again by renewing our vows. I did not know what to say for a few seconds and then of course said yes! It filled him with so much hope to be able to fantasize about how, where and when we were going to do it and he planned it out in his mind. It was bittersweet for me, wanting so much to see a recovery but at the same time I had kept a close watch on his liver tumors and I could feel them growing. We went all out in our fantasy about this wonderful second ceremony where it would be just Brian and me, with our two sons as witnesses. We have always liked it simple so when we got married 29 years ago it was just us and a friend as a witness.

He was so filled up with energy that we ended up sitting and working quite late that evening before going to bed. It was wonderful to see him energized in this way and it lasted for a bit over a month until his body started failing him again.

Day by Day
December 4, 2017

The days continue and my recovery from my healing does also. I long for the mundane things in life like going to the store, cooking, washing dishes…ok maybe not that. I take small steps like walking for five minutes a day, sitting up and doing what work I can. I've accomplished a lot by getting out three albums since this started… with a lot of help from friends of course. I long for spring and warmth and once again feel I might get there. It's slow going but I feel I'm getting there. Writing is still tiring, but it's more physical than mental. I say my mantra about purpose and keep my faith strong. It makes me so happy to hear that what I have written has inspired someone or led them to find their purpose. I have gotten so much love over the past months that I am truly humbled. Love is the heart of the world and life. Hold it dearly. Cherish your moments and share them with those you love.

Keep me in your prayers and thoughts. I love you all.
Brian

Happy Birthday to My Wife
December 5, 2017

My wife is a true source of strength to me. She spends the bulk of her time taking care of me. For that I love her, but that is not the only reason. Through this trial we have gotten so much closer, spent more time together and talk once again. I'm convinced that without her I would be dead by now. She's more beautiful than ever, both inside and out. Today is her birthday and I want to take this chance to let her know what she means to me.

In the bleak winter you are my light, my love and my strength

In the warm summer you are my sun

You are all the fragrances and promises of renewal in spring

In the autumn you add color to my life

I am grateful I found you once again for I have taken you for granted too much and too long

That will not happen again

I plan to love you, spend this life with you, and cherish our time together

I love you Fia, this song is for you.

LYING NEXT TO ME
music and lyrics by Brian Hobbs

Verse 1
Waiting for the night to fade
Wondering if the morning light will be my salvation
It gets harder to remember, all the things that made me smile
When I see all the dreams I've dreamed slowly fading
My one consolation,
You are here, lying next to me

Verse 2
Funny how we soon forget
Things that really mean the most are so seldom spoken
In the quest for our freedom we neglect the time to share
And so lives fall apart, and lives are mended
And through every disappointment
Every broken vow, every time I'm falling
Every time I'm down
My only consolation
You are here, lying next to me

Bridge
Giving me the reason to carry on
Making me feel like I still belong
And things will be alright
When my world starts to fall apart
You are there to heal my heart
Through every disappointment
Every broken vow
Every time I'm falling
Every time I'm down
My only consolation
You are here, lying next to me

It's the Journey

December 5, 2017

I look at dates and sometimes I wish I could go back in time but then I realize that I have changed so much. My entire outlook has changed, I see things so differently now. I have grown spiritually, emotionally and in my faith. One day at a time has become a reality. I see with different eyes now, more differently than I ever saw before. The transition has been hard and is still hard and I'm struggling in dealing with the day-to-day understanding of my condition. I want to recover and fulfill my purpose and I hope God allows me to do that. My world has changed drastically but I still feel positive and look forward to each new day. Like always, it's the Journey.

Please continue keeping me in your prayers.

Love, B.

Things I've Learned
December 6, 2017

The Christmas lights make our building and courtyard come alive this time of year. I love it. This will be a very special Christmas for me because, as I wrote yesterday, so much has changed. I can't do a lot physically so that is why I keep inundating you all with these posts. I think a lot and I watch people outside going about their everyday lives, the life I used to take for granted. Don't be like me, savor every moment, from going to school to buying groceries. You never know how much it all means until it is taken away. I'm not complaining, I've grown, and I think I'm a better person. I have a clarified purpose in life and hope I will get to use my newfound knowledge and spirituality to help others find their purpose. I know nothing I say here is new but it comes from my own experience and maybe that makes it unique.

Things I've learned:

Life is finite; use it, enjoy it, live it.
Family and friends are the most important things in this life.
Love means being there.

Love your spouse and children.
Finding your purpose is a gift.
Fulfilling your purpose is a bonus.

So at this time of year, remember the simple things, and love is the greatest of these. Create, share, love and embrace every aspect of this life while you can. Be someone's divine spark. Let God live in you and through you.

Please let me know your thoughts and continue to pray for my recovery.

Love to all, Brian.

Finding a Way—Good News
December 7, 2017

Sometimes things we want or need seem impossible, but other times a way is found, a door opens that you never knew existed. Call it faith, synchronicity, answered prayers, whatever. Today my liver and blood values had improved to 3.0 from 4.2 and 95 from around 83.

Small miracles, but miracles still the same. I'm glad, I'm thankful to God, I'm alive and kicking.

I know many prayers have been offered on my behalf and I just wanted to let you all know that it does work and I am forever grateful. Please keep them coming!

With love to all my divine sparks, B.

Fia's Reflections

The blood tests Brian was taking regularly were very important to him and I saw a big change in him every time he got a positive sign. For years this response has been called placebo but research shows that our thoughts communicate with our cells right down to our DNA level. Elizabeth Blackburn got the Nobel Prize in medicine 2009 about the subject of telomeres, the tiny ends on our DNA and how they age and wear down over time. The good news is they can also grow back with the help of stress management techniques like mindfulness which has been well-researched for more than 30 years. Candace Perth, a brain researcher who wrote the book Molecules of Emotion, established that the link between mind and body is our emotions that communicate with the cells through neuropeptides.

The body responds to your thoughts which creates emotions that affect your body and your immune system. By taking away hope you can block the natural healing response that happens in your body every day. Your body is constantly responding to all sorts of threats like viruses, bacteria, chemical poison and mutated cells among other things. It deals with it beautifully without us interfering until the day when your body has too much toxicity, chronic inflammation or mutated cells which causes your immune system to be under pressure. The first thing to turn it around would be to change the internal environment by avoiding food that has an inflammatory reaction in the body. What many people don't realize is that stress also has the same reaction on your body and by not dealing with the overpowering stress response you are putting your immune system out of balance so it cannot work the way it is supposed to.

It All Started with an Egg

December 9, 2017

*T*wo weeks ago, I wanted to die. I literally prayed for death. I met with my wife and children and asked them permission to let go and then said my goodbyes. But I didn't die. Luckily my prayer was not answered. And that weekend I lay in bed listening to my wife and children playing games and talking and laughing. I suddenly realized I didn't want to leave these people that I loved so much.

The whole dive had started because I was supposed to have an x-ray that week so we could see the size of the tumor. My oncologist cancelled it with the excuse of "what's the use?" I'm supposedly terminal and this was a confirmation. And as I lay in bed I realized, this woman doesn't know, she hasn't seen me in a month and no new x-rays have been taken since August. Plus she doesn't realize the power of prayer and all my divine sparks.

In the last two weeks my appetite has come back. I have probably gained a kilo and my liver value has improved to within 1 percentage point of normal.

The real change started on a Monday night, November 27. My entire family had gone to see my son perform in a play. My brother-in-law stayed with me. He was going to help with dinner, but his culinary skills are not the best so I got out of bed and fixed myself eggs and toast. I couldn't sleep so I ended up sitting up for 3 hours that night. After that everything changed. I started to live again.

I thank God and all of you for that miracle. All I know is new paths are opening and I am positive and believe. My wife is a rock and supports me endlessly. We are working hard and with your continued prayers another miracle might occur.

Just wanted to share this and thank you! Love, Brian

To My Wife

December 10, 2017

You, you come to me with a smile every day
You make me alive with your laugh
I never saw the sky until I looked in your eyes
I never felt the earth beneath my feet until you touched me
I never realized that love was tangible until you healed me
You are my strength, my cherished moment
You anoint me and I feel whole
I love you with all my heart.
Thank you for being you, for just being you.
I love you babe!

The Power of Divine Sparks

December 11, 2017

I feel blessed, which is a word that is much overused. The people praying for me, thinking of me and sending over strength and love are a big part of the recovery/healing process. It gives me the will to keep going, to have patience and to let things work in their own time. Sometimes it's hard to wait when you want recovery so badly, but your comments, Facebook likes, calls, messages and everything else give me peace and strength to keep on going.

It's one day at a time, but when you think about it, that's all we have; one day at a time, one minute, the very moment we live in is all we have.

My wife and I talked today about how everything negative evolves from fear. So why fear anything? Death is facing all of us so say hello to it, move on and live your life! It's easier than you think.

Please keep me in your prayers, anoint me with your comments and love and love one another and try to find your purpose. I am forever grateful.

Love, B.

Fia's Reflections

In one of our daily discussions Brian asked me how I saw and defined spirit. Brian was raised in a religious home and I was not. My own search and curiousness on life and its meaning started when I was 25. I read all kinds of books on the subject and also on death and dying. I really wanted to be able to find an answer that I could live with. One of the best questions that impacted my core beliefs was not about what happens when we die but what happens before we are born. Where do we come from? I figured it must be the same place we go back to when the body dies. One of my qigong masters put it in a way that I took to heart. He explained that we are all just little sparks, divine sparks, from the big fire that is the universe. We come from the universe and we go back to and become one with it. The same analogy goes for drops of water. We can part from the big ocean as a single drop but sooner or later we will reunite and be one out of many billions of water drops creating an ocean.

I believe that the life energy in us, the spark or spirit or whatever name you have for it, ignites us for a while on earth and then goes back to the main source to be charged again. People believe in different religions but if you peel away the words and the rituals, it is all about the spark of life that we still don't have a full understanding of. Whatever interpretation we put into it is fine if it can help us see the bigger picture and put things in perspective.

Visceral

December 11, 2017

There is something visceral about writing with a pen; the feel of the tip on the paper, holding the pen and moving it across the page. It's double work with the blog, but sometime I like doing it.

The same can be said of healing/recovery. By that I mean that if we savor everything associated with it; eating good, nutritional food, a little exercise, keeping the mind busy, meditation or prayer, etc., we feel the process. WE can't sit around waiting for God to do his work. WE have to "do". If things are bad for us then we have to make a change and stop. WE have to help God help us.

"Doing" is something visceral. We feel it. For someone like me, who is supposedly terminal, it passes the time of day, it gives you hope. You do what you can. Each thing we do today affects how we feel tomorrow. We have to move across the page of our lives just like a pen, otherwise we are not existing, not really living. Do what you can do no matter how small, live, don't exist. Remember, purpose is everything. If you need help, write me and I'll try to guide you. That is my God-given purpose. I am not fully recovered yet but I'll do what I can.

I love you all. Please keep visiting, reading, and sharing your comments.

B

Fia's Reflections

It was wonderful seeing him so determined to live his life no matter what and no matter how it would end. Every day when he woke up it was a new day. We ate breakfast together, I got him situated in the chair, he did some writing if he could, he slept, did some exercise, ate lunch, slept, the precious healing hour in the afternoon, maybe some writing again or a snooze, eating dinner if he could and then summing up the day. It was a good one, let's make tomorrow even better.

Thankful

December 13, 2017

A few weeks ago I was basically praying for death and I asked my sons and my wife for permission to let go. I wonder now how I could've ever done such a thing with people that I love and who I want to be with. It didn't take me long to realize how wrong I had been and I can't imagine living life without them or going into death and leaving them behind. I know I'll have to do it one day but not yet.

All that became apparent today as I was sitting in my chair watching the cold, dull, gray winter sky and all of a sudden, after taking a nap, I awoke to a beautiful snowfall and I cried because of the beauty in the world; not something I am ready to leave yet. I have learned to see beauty again in things that before I felt were a nuisance

I have simple pleasures planned for today. My wife is going to pick up food at a falafel place and we will enjoy that together for lunch later on. A dear friend is coming for dinner and fixing what he claims to be the world's best pancakes (THEY WERE). My son is here and the other son is coming home on the weekend. Life is good. I feel good. I still have no pain, which is amazing, and I'm relatively happy. My strength is still not what I want it to be but I'm working on that and things are moving in the right direction

I've resigned myself to the fact that I have cancer but I have not resigned myself to the fact that I will let it kill me. I will fight this thing with all my might, I will continue to pray, to love and to try and fulfill my purpose. A couple of months ago I could not see as far as Christmas. I thought without a doubt that I would be gone long before that but now as we approach it and are just a little more than two weeks away, I feel strong, I feel happy and I feel that this could be an amazing Christmas.

I am so thankful to God, to all my friends and all my divine sparks for everything you've done. Your prayers, thoughts and messages mean everything to me. Please continue to give me strength as I need all I can get.

Love, B

Divine Sparks are Flying!
December 15, 2017

There are two blog entries for today because it's been such an amazing 24 hours. I am so thankful for the generosity and love that everyone has sent to me by helping me almost meet my goal for my medical costs. I am truly humbled by this and amazed and consider it a true Christmas miracle. My journey to recovery started when I let go of all my fear. I think that fear is what feeds the cancer and what feeds many other illnesses in our bodies. I no longer fear death. I found my purpose, it's a God-given purpose, and for that I'm extremely thankful. I believe in miracles and I believe in change and I think that love heals, and that includes loving yourself.

Now I know that this is a recovery process, but I have already been healed, and I believe that with all my heart. Thank you all for believing in me, for believing in my purpose, and for giving me a chance to get this treatment that I so desire. I promise to keep you updated on my progress and I will try to write more blogs and put out more stories and hopefully stay in close contact with all of you. You truly are divine sparks.

Much love, Brian

Fia's Reflections

There was no curative treatment for Brian from the very beginning as the cancer was not detected until it was too late, all the symptoms he had were blamed on his heart problem. He was waiting for an operation of the heart but it dragged out until he was so sick that even the cardiologist started taking other tests. By that time the kidney tumor was 12 centimeters and protruding out of the left kidney, it had also spread to the liver.

We decided early on to focus on quality of life by nourishment, changing the diet and using CBD oil among other things. He also got hyperthermia and all of these things kept him free of pain until a few weeks before his death when he could no longer eat or get out of bed to get his treatments. I also worked hard to get high dose C-vitamin infusion but in Sweden the treatment is not accepted or easy to get hold of and we did not have the money to go anywhere to get it done. Brian's sister took it upon herself to start up a GoFundMe for Brian so people could help out with what he needed. We were both blown away by all the people sending money so we could continue what we did and save up for more treatments. He felt all the healing coming from friends and family and he opened up to receiving not just the money but the energy and thought behind it. It was a humbling experience for both of us and we counted ourselves the luckiest couple in the world. It would keep him alive for almost two more months.

Christmas Angels—a Story
December 15, 2017

I had been Christmas shopping in the city and was heading back home, tired, hungry and loaded down with bags and packages. They were both on the subway when I got on the train at Hötorget, two junkies; a man and a woman. She may have been pretty at one time; you could see that in the facial structure. But now her face was pallid and porous. She had a pasty complexion that showed all the bruises of time, even though she was much younger than she looked. She had the blank stare and jerky body language of someone who had been on the stuff for too long, surrendered herself to way too many men and spent much too long on the streets. She wore a dirty pink hat, old jeans, a man's oversized sweater and a ragged coat that couldn't possibly have kept out the cold of a Stockholm winter. Her companion looked to be in worse shape; a large, rough looking, unshaven man devoid of life, one of the walking dead. She was talking to the man; loudly and incoherently, gesticulating with her jerky movements, and like the scared, hunted animals you see on those television nature programs, her dark eyes never focused or rested on any one object too long. They flitted back and forth

113

all the time like she was constantly on the lookout for an attacker, for danger, trying to avoid the beatings, robberies and rapes she'd probably suffered during her years on the street.

At the next station a group of high-school kids got on and sat in the seats across from her and her junkie boyfriend. The girls in this group were the polar opposites of this woman; young, happy, well-off and pretty. From the equipment they were carrying you could tell they had been ice-skating in Kungsträdgården. Some of the girls still carried their skates in their hands.

"How much does a pair of skates cost?" asked the junkie girl to no one in particular.

There was no answer. The other girls just kept talking and laughing.

"How much does a pair of skates cost today?" the junkie girl asked again.

She must have thrown this question out there four or five times before she got an answer from one of the girls.

"A good pair will cost about 600 crowns."

The junkie girl's facial expression did not change at all. She just looked back at the girl, shook her head and repeated "600 crowns." She stared at the girl and said in a jagged, fragile voice, "I used to skate when I was a girl in Bulgaria. I was very good."

By that time the train was at the next stop and the high-school kids bounced off, the girls still laughing and talking about whatever it is that high-school girls talk about. But just before the subway doors closed, one of the girls turned around, looked at the junkie girl, held out her skates and said "take these, they look like they'll fit you". Then she smiled and ran off the train.

The junkie girl sat there, holding the pair of skates, not really registering the gift, when suddenly her lifeless eyes sparkled as tears started running down her face. She clutched those skates like they were the most precious things in the world, and maybe those skates were her "ruby slippers". Maybe they transported her far away to a place called home because then a glow came back to that waxen complexion. And in her tears I saw a world of hurt and bad decisions get washed away and I felt like I could look inside her mind and see a little girl in Bulgaria, floating and gliding over the ice: free, warm, safe and loved. And for the first time in what I imagine was a very long time, she smiled. Not that fake, forced junkie smile to try to entice someone into giving her the next fix, but the smile of a child, content and filled with wonder, hope and amazement.

I got off at the next stop but the junkie girl and her boyfriend stayed on. And as I walked down the platform I felt uplifted, like I'd witnessed a Christmas miracle, and I prayed and hoped with all my heart that another angel would come along and take that girl skating so that she could experience the joy that I imagined I saw in her mind.

The following week I was at a Christmas party in town and it was filled with the usual cross-section of Stockholmers; people from Östermalm, Södermalm, Saltsjöbaden, Lidingö and Kungsholmen all talking about finances, the prices of apartments and houses, art and music, their kids, television shows and movies. I was standing in a group and one of the men started talking about how he had taken his kids to the skating rink and seen a young homeless woman standing outside carrying around a pair of what looked to be very expensive ice skates.

"What an odd thing for a homeless person to be carrying around," someone said.

"They wouldn't let her in because of the way she was dressed, the way she looked. I intervened since it was Christmas, I wanted to be an example to my girls, so I shamed the rink attendant into letting her get in. It was like I had given her a winning lottery ticket. I've never gotten so many 'thank yous' in my life. I watched her skate and she was actually quite good at it."

He and everyone else were surprised when I started to laugh and cry at the same time. He was especially surprised when I gave him a hug. This flood of emotion came over me and in my mind I could see the junkie girl I'd seen on the subway flying across the ice, graceful and swanlike, doing spins and figure eights, smiling. And I knew that at least for those few moments, she was free, she was happy and she was young again, overtaken by the innocence she'd lost so long ago.

People were asking me what was wrong and I wiped my eyes and said, "I know people talk a lot about angels at Christmastime, and I have to be honest and say I never really believed in them…until now. In the last week I've seen two with my own eyes."

Christmas is Coming

December 16, 2017

I feel so lucky today because I have both my boys home. They're decorating the tree and fixing things for the holidays, it's wonderful to have them here.

As I watch them decorate the tree I'm reminded of many Christmases when I was young. My father would take us driving around to look at all the Christmas lights in town. Most of the Christmas decorations were extremely gaudy, but as a child I was enamored with the whole thing. We would stop by my grandmother's house where we loaded up on Coca-Cola, Hershey's kisses, and fruit cake for my dad.

I remember looking under the tree at all the beautifully wrapped packages and hoping with all my heart that there was something in there for me. It was all I could do not to touch them.

I'm also happy to be here, just to be here. Almost three weeks ago I was on my deathbed, I was ready to die. But somehow I came back through God's love, and through the love of my family I was drawn out of the depths and brought back to life and things have been improving ever since. I'm still quite weak and it takes all my strength to do these blogs and just to get through the simple everyday things I have to do. The will to live is a wonderful thing. Love is what saved me. No other medicine comes close to it

Here is a nice song for you for third Advent. It's sung by Johan Becker and we also wrote it together. Hope you enjoy it!

Fia's note: The song Christmas Is Coming has not been released officially.

Fia's Reflections

Brian had bought tickets to A Soulful Christmas months ago. It is an annual Christmas concert with his songwriting partner Andreas Aleman and a band, singing and playing original songs by Brian and Andreas as well as traditional Christmas carols. At this point Brian was not able to go but wanted me to take one of our sons and enjoy the evening. I was filming it for him so he could see it from his bed at home. It was bittersweet to be at the concert without Brian but I knew he took pride in these concerts and wanted us to be there.

Goals

December 17, 2017

*T*he world changed when I got cancer. I had to change with it. The positive thing is that I found my faith again. After lying, waiting for death, I was healed. And I'm waiting for recovery instead. I looked at a list of goals that I wrote back in September.

They were:

Live to see my boy's graduate college.
Put out my albums.
Gain weight.
Say goodbye to those I love.
Not lose my faith.

I did lose my faith briefly but now it's stronger than ever. I did say goodbye to my loved ones, but I also said goodbye to fear of death and dying. I put out my albums. My new goals have become:

Cancer-free in 2018.
Life.
Purpose.
Helping others.
It's the journey, folks. I'm learning, I'm alive, and I'm loving. Life
is good.

Bless you all.
Brian

Truly Random Thoughts
December 18, 2017

*T*oday I'm tired. Yesterday was a good day and I probably overdid it. My mantra is that I'm already healed and that this is the recovery. It's hard but life is worth it and I'm blessed to be here for another day. I'm sorry my writing is not so eloquent anymore. I mostly use a dictating program to write these blogs so the sentences tend to be shorter. I take indoor walks because I can't really get out. I also got an exercise bike today that we have to put together so I hope we can manage that, then I can hopefully strengthen my legs. Other than that I'm sitting up more. I don't go to bed during the day, I don't lie down, which is good, so I consider all and all things are improving.

I feel so thankful for everything because honestly, I never imagined that I would still be here on December 18. It's less than ten days until Christmas Eve and I'm looking forward to having all my family at home and getting together with relatives for some excellent Swedish Christmas food. My sister-in-law makes something called Jansson's temptation which is delicious. I'm really looking forward to that.

As you can see my life is made up of small moments and in small hopes, but this is what keeps me going during the day. My next goal is to make it into 2018. I really never believed one or two months ago that I would make it that far but now I have hope.

As I guess many of you have noticed there's been a change in my life during this ordeal. The most important thing is that I have regained my faith and renewed my spirituality. I don't wear my beliefs or religion on my sleeve and I think that a man should be judged by his actions rather than his beliefs. As I've written before I know I have a purpose in this life and I pray that God will allow me to fulfill that purpose. It makes me feel very good when I can fulfill my purpose even now, and I hear that people are inspired by things I write. I'm still amazed by the outpouring of love from all of you. It brings me both joy and humbles me.

I'll continue rambling for a while if you let me. I do believe in miracles and I am expecting one with my situation. I ask for your continued prayers and that you keep me in your thoughts. You are a true blessing and I love you all.

The world is strange, it's strange that I still have this incredible desire to express myself. I know I'm rambling again but, these are random thoughts.

I am at peace. And this peace gives me something to live for, something to work towards, and a real goal for fulfilling my purpose, which right now is the most important thing in the world for me.

It's a time of love and miracles right now so I hope we can all remember to celebrate the season and celebrate the reason. For me, there is no Christmas stress. There are no gifts to buy because of money constraints in our house right now. That's actually quite refreshing. We just plan on enjoying being with each other, eating good food and celebrating the season in the way it was meant to be celebrated as the season of love and miracles.

I can probably keep talking for a long time but I better end this thing, I love you all and I continue to ask for your prayers and I thank you for everything you've given me, all the love you've sent me. I will probably be posting more as we get close to the holidays and possibly presenting one or two of my stories which I hope you will like. If you like the stories I hope you'll consider donating to my Go Fund me account which is now underway. As you may have read earlier we have unexpected medical expenses and need help in covering these. Thank you for whatever you can give. Your donations are much appreciated, they will be used for a good cause. Merry Christmas for now and love to you all.

Brian.

Thanks and a Quick Update!

December 19, 2017

Once again I want to thank everyone who has contributed to my GoFundMe account. We have raised over 6,000 dollars!!!!! Thank you and bless everyone who has been so generous.

I have started exercising more to try to strengthen my body. It's tough and after my 15 minutes I'm very tired, so I don't do much else. But like Fia says, sometimes you get to play the C-card as an excuse.

I'm amazed how much my body has changed. I actually tried to play the piano for the first time in 5 months. Not good…I will have to relearn all the muscle movements, plus I never imagined my fingers would become so weak. Other than that my appetite is good, I do what I can do and I am getting bored, which Fia says is a good sign. Speaking of Fia, she is still my angel, sacrificing her own work to take care of me. I'm truly fortunate and blessed.

I know it's a busy time of year but please let me hear from you. It brings me joy and hope and I still need my divine sparks to keep me in thoughts and prayers.

I'm sure I'll be writing over the holidays so we'll speak soon. Love to all! Brian

A Christmas Prayer

December 20, 2017

Dear God,

I thank you for letting me be alive today, for all the small things I can do. I thank you for your healing and now I ask that you carry me through my recovery.

I thank you for all the divine sparks you've given me and for the prayers and thoughts and the generosity and people. I thank you for taking away my fear of death, and for giving me hope.

I thank you for changing me and defining my purpose. I pray you will let me fulfill that purpose.

I thank you for my wife and children, friends and relatives and others who have come into my life. I thank you for my students who have shown so much love.

I thank you for Christmas and all it means. I never expected to be alive or even be here to see this day much less for Christmas.

I especially thank you for my two sons who've been a great inspiration to me and been a great help as well. Without them, I seriously doubt I would be here today.

I am so thankful for so many things, but these are some of the more specific things I wanted to thank you for. Thank you for the tender mercies of generous people, they have given so much and give me so much hope.

I guess most of all I thank you for giving me back my faith, something that I had let slide many, many years ago. And now I pray for peace, love and understanding in this world, something we desperately need. I also pray that you let me be a part of achieving that goal.

Thank you for everything God and please send your love to all my divine sparks.

When the Tree is Green Again

December 21, 2017

*T*here's a tree outside the room where my wife gives me hyper-thermia treatments. It has become a metaphor for my tumor. Right now it is cold and ugly, with scraggly limbs and branches like claws. This is my tumor, trying to hold on, grasping at me claw-like. But in a few months this tree will be green, soft and lush. Today I decided that I will see this tree green again. It will have released its grasp and become another part of me.

Life changes and I have to hold on until the claws let go and the warmth comes again.

God is good. I have my dark moments when the claws reach out, but overall I'm positive, and just as spring is a miracle, I expect my recovery to be the same.

Please send strength and prayers. Love to all! Merry Christmas.

Brian

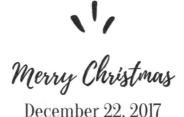

Merry Christmas
December 22, 2017

One month ago I was lying on my deathbed praying for death. Today I am still here looking forward to Christmas with my family. I feel I'm getting stronger, from general health indications my tumor is not growing or spreading. Prayers have been answered and I believe.

It's nothing short of a miracle. Miracles are real, I have seen too many now not to believe. I am still weak but very much alive. Here is a Christmas gift to all my divine sparks. Please continue to pray. It means so much to me and it WORKS!

It's a lullaby to the Christ child. I hope you enjoy it. The words I wrote have taken on a new meaning for me now.

Merry Christmas to all!

GO TO SLEEP from Brian Hobbs's album Candle in the Window, sung by Mia Löfgren, can be found on Spotify.

What is Christmas?

December 24, 2017

For me, it's God's love sent down from above
It's the joy in our hearts and from those we love
It's the magic and wonder we often forget
It's the miracle we can't see or haven't seen yet
It's the awakening of the senses, a turning to the light
A star in the darkness lighting the night
It's kindness and hope, charity and prayer
It's knowing your divine sparks are always there

Prayer Does Change Things

December 27, 2017

*Y*esterday I watched a very interesting DVD that scientifically proved that we are all connected and that our beliefs and feelings actually change things in our world. That pretty much translates into prayer changes things. I knew that but it's interesting to get a scientific take on things. Since I regained my faith I have known that all these divine sparks are real and important. That is why I appreciate each and every one of you. I started my recovery exactly one month ago today.

I truly believe and feel that God has healed me and am only waiting for the tumor to disappear. I know that this feeling is due to all the prayers from all of you. I ask that you continue to keep me in your thoughts and keep anointing me with your prayers. I have been called to a new purpose that I will talk about later. I will say that it involves purpose and healing. I hope I get to share with you. Much love to all! Remember, there is love and fear. Choosing love is choosing life. Fear is the path to despair.

Happy New Year!
December 31, 2017

I am sitting here with my family listening to music while they cook dinner. Cancer fatigue wears me down but I am grateful to be here. 2017 has been the year from hell for me, but I'm alive, I still have a chance and much to be thankful for. There is always the dichotomy, the bad with the good. I never imagined myself in this situation, but I am a changed man. I have regained my faith, been given so much love and had my purpose defined. I have said goodbye to my fear of death and have chosen life. I struggle, but I'm still here to continue recovery and live up to becoming cancer-free in 2018. I have so many people who love me and care. I am truly blessed. Thank you all for your support over these last months. I know I would not be here without you.

I wish everyone a great year and send you all my love. In Sweden, please remember to be kind to the animals that suffer so much from the fireworks. Let the fireworks come from inside you and send love out instead of noise. Love to all and Happy New Year!

Love,

Brian

Fia's Reflections

We were all amazed that Brian was able to be with us over Christmas and New Year. He was tired but did put in five minutes exercise on his bike and he walked inside the house for ten minutes on Christmas day. He no longer had the strength to do the stairs in the hallway and it was too cold for him to be outside. He was constantly cold even inside and had blankets and a heater on most of the time.

We had a pre-New Year's dinner on the 29th for the whole family including my sister and brother-in-law and on the 31st it was just Brian, me, our two sons and one of our son's girlfriend. It meant so much for all of us to be together that night as we knew it would be the last New Year's Eve. Brian stayed up until midnight, had a sip of champagne and then went to bed, ready to face 2018.

Another Day

January 2, 2018

This is my therapy so I really appreciate people reading my random thoughts. It's difficult writing because of cancer fatigue, but your comments and being able to share with you is what keeps me going. Another breakdown today, like a pendulum between despair and thankfulness for being alive. I cry a lot more than I ever have. Fia says that's natural.

But I am still able to eat and sleep. Still able to write although it is difficult. I am waiting to see when my treatment can start. I am hoping the last week of this month latest. I am still eternally grateful to everyone who contributed to the GoFundMe account and contributed in other ways. I am grateful for many things, especially the support and love I get from all of you. It's a lifeline. I'd especially like to thank Arnold Wiley for constantly offering up prayers on my behalf and for other cancer sufferers. There are many others who keep me in their prayers and I love all of you too.

I wish I had more words of wisdom or insights to share but I don't. I must remind myself that love is all there is; I must keep believing that through my faith and beliefs, recovery is coming; I must believe that there is a divine plan and that I have a purpose to fulfill. I must stay positive. There is so much I have yet to do and my purpose is clear now. Please pray that I am granted the strength to carry it out.

I am not a strong person but I have many around me giving me strength to carry on. Love is life and true life is love. Even in my darkest hour there is light. I just have to focus on that. I guess we all do.

Thanks again for reading. It means more than you know. Keep the comments coming. Love to you all.

Brian

Waiting for a Miracle

January 3, 2018

*T*oday has been a strange day. I woke up feeling as if my tumor was gone. Of course it's still there but it was an affirmation of my healing. I know that through God's grace one day it will be gone. I stay busy working on my songwriting book and just recovering. Good days and bad days and sometimes a mix in between. Things are moving the right way with treatment and I hope I can start soon. Everyday takes me closer to my miracle. I truly believe that. I have ups and downs and will continue to have them. But I am trying to hold onto my faith.

Love is still the miracle.

Fia's Reflections

Being able to be thankful in a situation like this takes a lot of courage, strength and faith. It is much easier to fall into the role of victimhood and sink deep into depression. I think somehow that when you are close to losing it all, you start appreciating the little things you take for granted and every little positive change becomes a miracle. I think it is about self-preservation and I saw so many examples with Brian where the smallest things could lift him out of his dark days. It would give him an energy boost and a sense of purpose. The placebo effect is a strong force to be reckoned with as it lifts both body and spirit.

The Craft of Creating is Now Available as an eBook

January 3, 2018

Fia's Reflections

Brian had been working as a singer-songwriter teacher at a school nearby called Kulturama. He truly enjoyed teaching and encouraging the students to find their own voice and style in their writing. He was much loved and there were many students who came by and sent messages, flowers etc.

He had lots of material that he had written that was used as a textbook but he had not had the time to put it together in a book. I helped him get it sorted and after much work I got it done and it was uploaded as an eBook on Amazon. This was done on January 3rd and was a big relief for Brian to finally get it out there. He felt an immense sense of purpose and fulfillment at being able to leave something behind to inspire songwriters to find their purpose and voice.

Boredom and Recovery

January 4, 2018

The boredom of just waiting for recovery has set in. Since June I have put out four albums, one single and a book. It was all bucket list stuff. I have started on a book about my experiences with cancer and my healing and recovery. Yes, I believe I'm healed. God has done that, and I truly believe. It is not apparent yet but through all the love it will become so. The recovery is taking time. That's what my faith tells me.

I feel compelled to share my story and have a purpose to help others find their purpose. Patience has never been one of my virtues, so maybe this is another of my lessons. I have already regained my faith and learned to let love decide.

I pray for recovery and my greatest desire is to serve others in the future. I feel I have a lot to give. My flesh is weak but I feel my spirit growing stronger and I have to express that by pecking out this blog one finger style.

Please continue to pray that I will find the strength to continue on my journey and hopefully help someone along the way. Let me say I certainly don't have it all figured out but I sincerely hope someone is comforted or inspired by my words and thoughts. Thanks again for reading and responding. It means the world to have these connections with my divine sparks. Let love guide you!

Brian

Fia's Reflections

Brian wanted to be able to share his experiences and give other people hope and encourage them to face their fears and move past them. He wanted to give talks together with me and speak about the different healing stages and that it is not only the physical healing that is important. True healing comes from within and has to happen on an emotional, mental and spiritual level and if the physical body is still able, then it is the last level for healing to take place. Having a strong purpose can help you get very far.

Prayer, Meditation and Rambling
January 5, 2018

I am praying and meditating tonight. As you know I run the gamut between despair and hope. But deep in my soul I know that God is working. He changed me and changed my purpose.

I believe that God is in every one of us. I feel that love, God's love, is the same as our love, which He moves through us.

There are so many things I have yet to do. I want to help people discover healing and their purpose in life. I hope you believe that's not out of some selfish desire to live, but of a genuine desire to serve.

Anyway, I just wanted to clarify. My heart and mind are clear for the moment and I feel blessed to have such a wonderful wife and children. Fia, Adam and Jeremy, I love you immensely. I am grateful for all the prayers and thoughts from my divine sparks. You are all wonderful. I am grateful that I have gotten to see 2018. I am ready to recover and do my work. Please keep me in your prayers. I know I ask a lot and this takes time, but please keep the love and prayers coming. I need them now more than ever.

A quick update…I hope to start my treatment in the next week or so and it will continue for two weeks and then we will evaluate the results. Thanks again to everyone who donated. I am forever grateful.

Well, this has been part of my meditation and I will continue with my prayer. Love to you all, and to my friends in North Carolina, be careful in all that snow. Please write me, even just to say hi. I love hearing from you. I apologize for rambling on.

Love, Brian

The Room and Healing

January 6, 2018

I wasn't going to write today but felt compelled to. I wanted to talk about the treatment room where my wife and I go for her treatment one hour a day. It's a safe room, meaning that I can cry, express what I'm feeling and be free without worrying about looking weak or seeming like I'm complaining. Plus, she and I talk and she gives me comfort.

Everyone suffering from cancer needs this, a personal place to lay things out. This is one of the most important hours of my day. I get in touch with God in this room, or at least feel much closer.

In following my purpose, I also wanted to remind all that healing comes from inside. We sometimes forget and expect God to do all the work. He has the power but we have to take the initiative, whether physical or emotional healing. Prayer changes things, but so do we. Make changes in your life, follow HIS plan not yours. I am still struggling with this so I speak from experience.

I don't have the answers, but I'm learning patience, love, trust and faith every day. Once again, it's the journey. Please pray for me as I continue on mine.

Love, Brian

Fia's Reflections

Today Brian found more music on his computer that he made years ago. It is all instrumental and he wanted to get it out as soon as possible so we sat up and worked late.

He wanted me to name the 4 pieces and also the album so it became Healing Purpose and can be found on CD baby at the following link: https://store.cdbaby.com/cd/brianhobbs12

The instrumentals are called: *The Healing Room, Letting Go, Finding Purpose and Love is All There is*. Although he did not have energy to remaster them, they are beautiful pieces and I am glad he wanted to put them out as they were.

For Björn—Lesson Learned

January 7, 2018

A reprise from a year ago when my pup, Rusty, passed over (January 21, 2017).

I had a heavy heart this morning and out of habit I got dressed and prepared to go outside. Until yesterday this was my morning ritual; my walk with Rusty. It didn't matter to him whether it was sunny, raining, snowing, hot or cold.

We had to say goodbye to Rusty yesterday after 16 years of being together. In honor of his memory I decided to continue my walk this morning, but not just any walk. I decided to retrace the steps I have taken so many times before with him; I revisited his favorite places.

I cried. I laughed. My heart broke again and was healed a little when the sunlight broke through just like it did when he died yesterday. I think it will be this way for a very long time.

On my solitary walk the main thing that struck me was that Rusty was not one for sticking to the walking paths. He went his own way. And at the time I would get so frustrated with him because he would drag me over slippery patches of ice, knee-deep snow, ankle-deep mud, through puddles and weeds and high water. And it didn't really hit me until today that the paths, while easy to navigate, and safer, don't always hold the wonders of what lies just beyond. And I smiled because I realized that my little dog was still teaching me things.

I can only imagine what led Rusty off the paths to the magic and joy he found there, or if he really found anything at all. Maybe it was just a "dog thing". I don't know.

But it did make me think, and when I take the time to think I usually end up writing one of these…

Fia's note: Rusty was our beloved dog, a wire haired dachshund that came into our lives in the end of year 2000. On January 21, 2017 we took him to the vet to give him his final rest.

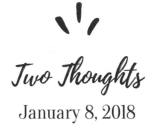

Two Thoughts

January 8, 2018

I woke up with two questions in my head today:
What purpose does worry serve?
What healing does worry accomplish?
Please think about it
Love,
Brian

Fia's Reflections

Brian got a walker today from the occupational therapist so he can walk more safely indoors and also out in the hallway. His muscles have deteriorated and he no longer trusts himself to walk alone. I do not allow him to get up at night alone at this stage and I help him every night to get to the bathroom. I also help him with showers and everything else he needs.

God Is in All of Us and We Are All Connected

January 9, 2018

God is in all of us and all of us are connected. I am reminded of this not only by my own Bible but by what my wife just read in the Tao (the book of Tao Te Ching).

We are born from God and return to God. I know all this is deep but I feel God moving through me today, not only with a healing power but with enlightenment. I hope that people won't be turned off by all this talk about God. I am not turning into a fanatic. It's just the easiest designation for what I feel is the divine spirit.

I have been blessed with an awakening and just want to share it. It really has more to do with purpose than religion. My purpose is to help others find their purpose, I know that now. Whether they want to learn to write songs and create or just become more aware. Each of us has a purpose. Finding out what that purpose is might take some guidance. If God allows, that is my purpose, to show others the way to their own purpose through His help.

Again, I hope this helps someone along the way to search out their purpose and find it. Life is so much more fulfilling once you have a purpose. Even with cancer I am trying to fulfill my own purpose. I am believing in a full recovery so that I can continue and hopefully help others.

Please continue to pray for me. Love,

Brian

Fia's Reflections

Brian expressed his new spirituality that he had discovered by calling it God or a divine spirit and everyone around him were divine sparks. We had many philosophical discussions and today I read Tao Te Ching for him as that is my spiritual book and has been for over 30 years. He was interested in hearing about different angles and could see the common ground for many religions around the world. I told him a story I heard about religion being like a banana peel. It can look different on the outside but inside you will find the golden nugget of spirituality, the banana itself.

By now he is dictating his blogs to me and I write them out for him. He has started C-vitamin infusions but I could tell it was way too late and he should have had them much earlier back in September. It is not easy to get it done in Sweden but I finally got it set up. There was a sudden change in him for the better but the cancer was too far spread to make a difference. He has started going to bed during the days now which is not a good sign.

To say I was tired was an understatement. I was getting myself ready for the end and I had no idea how much time we had left together. This was to become his last blog entry.

The Second Time We Almost Lost Him

January 13, 2018

*T*oday was the second time we almost lost him, the first time being November 23. The whole family gathered and we sat with him all day. In the midst of all this my brother got diagnosed with lung cancer. I am getting used to having a bunch of bad things happen all at once. Last time it happened was in 2010 when Brian got thyroid cancer. The same week he was diagnosed my colleague died of cancer and one of my best friends got diagnosed with lung cancer. She died four years later. That whole week was and still is a blur to me.

Tough Weekend

January 14, 2018

*I*t has been a tough weekend and Brian has started to take morphine for his pain in the liver and to be able to get more peaceful rest. Up until now he has not been in pain so I could tell that the end was coming closer. It is very hard to watch someone you love waste away in front of you. He was no longer able to get out of bed at all. My sister came up to keep me company and stayed for a few days to help out. I remember us cleaning out the kitchen. It was therapeutic for me as there was not much else I could do and it kept me busy when I was not helping Brian.

On January 19 Brian got a catheter put in place which was a big help to me and I did not have to get up at nights with him. That same evening one of our sons had his first gig and I was able to go because Andreas came and spent the evening with Brian. Although Brian was too tired to speak he appreciated having Andreas there but at the same time sad to show how sick he was. Not wanting to upset people was so typical of Brian.

Stopped Eating

January 20, 2018

*T*oday Brian stopped eating. Before he had maybe tasted a bite of something but from today he only wanted to drink water. I honored his wish as I know this is not unusual when you reach the end. The body cannot deal with digesting food when it is so weak. I thought he had his mind set on dying the next day.

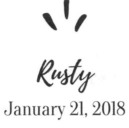

Rusty

January 21, 2018

A year ago today we had to put our beloved dachshund to sleep. He was 16 years and 3 months and he meant the world to all of us. Brian was hit really hard by the loss and I had to convince him that it was time for Rusty to let go. We all went to the vet but when it came time to give Rusty the final shot, Brian left the room. I sat with the dog together with my sons and we talked to him and patted him and he left so peacefully. It was a good closure to his long and happy life.

Not surprisingly, Brian got his third close to death experience today and his breathing was really bad. Both our sons and I were sitting with him and all he wanted to do was to fall asleep for good he said. That did not happen and he had two more tough days where he had to be given a sedentary injection. After those intense three days and nights I was totally exhausted, waiting for him to draw his last breath. I was by his side constantly, sleeping together with him in our bed although there was not much sleeping on my part. I wanted to be there all the time so he could reach for me whenever. Knowing I was there made him feel safe.

Holding out for Something

January 27, 2018

*T*oday Brian has been without food for seven days. After he drank some water and I had washed his face with a facial cloth he asked about today's date. I told him and I had a feeling he was holding out for something and reminded him that we had met 30 years ago on January 30. He remembered it well he said.

After his five close to death experiences on November 23 and January 13, 21, 22, 23 he had a calm week.

Thirty Years
January 30, 2018

*B*rian has been coughing a few nights and I have not been able to sleep. I look and feel as bad as him right now. I cooked a nice fish soup and had some champagne to celebrate our 30 years together but for Brian it was the tenth day with no food. He was aware though and was happy he survived the date. I thought he would be able to let go by now but he was still hanging on.

Nursing Team
February 2, 2018

Today we decided that the nursing team would come on a regular basis to help me out as it was getting harder each day to care for Brian. I needed help with turning him a few times a day and on February 3 they gave him a morphine pump so we could regulate on our own when he needed it. The nurses came by three times a day from now on to help me. It felt good to get the help but I still slept next to Brian and heard his every breath and cough. I was exhausted but did not want to leave his side. He stopped drinking water today and from now on, instead of counting days I counted hours. I was up all night.

Stuck in the House

February 3, 2018

14 days without food. I do not leave the house and my sister came by with groceries.

World Cancer Day

February 4, 2018

*T*oday is World Cancer Day and I usually attend it every year. This year I did not dare to leave the house. We were all home and took turns in sitting with Brian. I played music for him softly and friends came over with food and we ate together. Feels like he will pass over today.

Intense

February 5, 2018

*E*very hour is like the last for Brian, intense. Today is my in-law's 63rd wedding anniversary.

Unstable

February 6, 2018

Four days without water, not stable and thought he would die this afternoon.

Pain

February 7, 2018

*F*ive days without water, irregular breathing and short stops, I listen to every breath and sit close to him so he can feel that I am here. When the nurse came to turn him tonight it was the first time he showed pain and he got more morphine. His lungs made a rattling noise like they never had before and I could hear deep sighs. From 1.30 a.m. it calmed down and we both got to sleep the rest of the night.

Brian's Last Day

February 8, 2018

Sixth day with no water and 19 days without food. How is that even possible? Around 10.45 his breathing became almost effortless and hardly noticeable. I sat on the bed together with my son, his girlfriend and of course our dog Lucy who seemed to know what was up. We sat there for the next hour with Brian, listening to his breathing becoming softer until we could not even hear him. It was peaceful with no dramatic last sigh, he just slowly and quietly slipped over to the other side. This last hour he looked peaceful even though the disease and the past weeks had been rough on him. We sat there and talked to him and to each other until we could no longer feel his pulse and the heart stopped beating. It was sad but a tremendous relief for him and for us as the past three weeks had been taking a toll on my health as well.

We called the doctor and the nurse came and prepared him for the last ride. The doctor said that it was his strong heart that had made it possible for him to hang on so long which to me was incredible as he had major heart problems for the past three years before the cancer. Up until the ambulance came we were fine, he was there in the room with us and we felt at peace that he had finally let go. When the men came to pick him up and put him in a black plastic bag was when I totally broke down. Even writing about it now makes me tear up and it is a very hard image to block out. To see the person you love and have cared for be taken out in a black bag is something I never want to experience again. I understand why it is necessary but it is a memory and an image stuck in my mind that I have had to deal with for many months.

A few months earlier Brian had expressed that he was hoping to die in his sleep. "How would that feel?" I asked. "Great!" he said.

The Following Days

*H*ow people react after a loss is different. Some go into depression and cannot get anything done. Some busy themselves. I am one of those who takes control and starts working; that is my way of dealing with tragedy. The same night Brian died I was cleaning out shoes and clothes. What to get rid of and what to give away. Both sons and my sister were there and we all got busy.

The day after I started looking into funeral services.

I took a long walk with my dog for the first time in months. My son had taken care of her as I had not been able to leave the house and I felt a tremendous sense of freedom in the midst of all the grief. I noticed I had lost my stamina and was huffing as I walked up some stairs and a hill.

On February 12, I got a message from a man in New York saying that he will perform a song live that Brian had written the lyrics to.

I slowly eased back to work on February 13. I saw my first patient and the same night I held my regular qigong class for my students. Looking back it seems unreal but I was ready to busy myself and had to do something.

February 14 would have been our 29th wedding anniversary. I was not sure how to deal with it so my sister came over. We had the day off and went to a beautiful art exhibition that I know Brian would have loved. I could feel his presence with me. Afterwards we went to a restaurant and celebrated the years I have had with Brian.

There was a memorial service held for Brian on February 17 in his hometown in North Carolina and about one hundred people showed up. Brian had put together the music he wanted to be played. Unfortunately I could not be there as I was in the midst of planning for the funeral and the Swedish memorial service. We held a small funeral service for family only on March 16th at the columbarium where his ashes reside. It was a cold day and we had candles, flowers and his picture together with the urn. We played Brian's songs and when it was time to bring the urn to the grave we did it to the music of Jobim and Agua de Marco, a song that meant a lot to both us and always helps to lift my spirit.

The Swedish memorial took place in Stockholm on April 21. Close to a hundred people came and there were live performances of Brian's songs from his songwriting friends. There was so much heart and love that afternoon. Both me and my sons were exhausted afterwards and could not do anything for the rest of the weekend. I felt as if I had been through a tumble dryer and had just stepped out.

From here on the following months were filled with more practicalities that had to be dealt with and it took quite a while before I could take the time and deal with my grief. It is now, a year later, I feel I have caught up with my life again and started to look ahead.

Conversations with Brian

These are some of the topics that Brian and I talked about in the healing room during his healing hour. I have condensed them to the core.

Disbelief

For a long time Brian could not take in that he had stage 4 cancer, he just did not grasp it. It was not pure denial but more disbelief. I knew immediately what it meant but kept it to myself and mobilized my strength into taking action to give him the best quality of life.

Purpose

The finding of purpose was important to Brian and gave him a strong mission. This was Brian's mantra:

I have a purpose, God gave me this purpose, I know my purpose,
My purpose is to help other people find their own purpose.

I encourage you to find your own mantra that will help you in moments of despair and that will give you a strong sense of purpose.

Healing

We went for a proactive approach from day one. Focusing on living instead of not dying. Focusing on what Brian could do and not on what he couldn't. We started our healing hour every afternoon in my clinic room where we had long talks and he got healing treatments for anxiety and he worked his way through fear. The most profound healing happens on an emotional, mental and spiritual level and that can speed up the healing of the physical body. Sometimes physical healing is not possible but to reach healing on the other levels helps you go through the transition of death with an easier heart and without anxiety.

Diet

It took two cancer diagnoses for Brian to realize he could not go on with his diet of drinking coke, eating candy and unhealthy food in general. It was hard for him to kick his sugar habit and at the same time working as hard as he did gave him no time for exercise. On the other hand he never had an interest in exercise. Once he got the second and final cancer it all changed overnight. He was open and willing to eat healthy and had no problems quitting sugar. In fact he became an advocate of healthy eating and could not understand why he did not do it years earlier.

Rediscovery of Self

Brian's rediscovery of himself led to him finding out what was most important in life to him. Aside from his family it was letting go of fear, regaining spirituality and faith, belief in a higher power and believing in miracles again. There are so many things and values in life that will change a person forever after being diagnosed with a life-threatening disease. You come out as a changed person and that goes for the people close by as well.

Accepting and Preparing for Death

Once Brian realized his cancer was terminal he prepared for his memorial service, both the one in the States and the one that took place in Stockholm. He planned the music to be played and who was going to perform live on stage. He looked death in the face and made plans, after that he choose life and cherished it for as long as he had it.

Learning to Receive

Gifts, flowers, warm support and kind words of love were showered over Brian when he was still alive. That was such a blessing to witness. To be on the receiving end can put you in a vulnerable position but we felt that all the support was given with so much love and it was quite overwhelming to take it all in at times. Close to the end I had to read all the messages that came regularly to Brian as he was too tired to read them himself. We laughed and we cried together and felt humble for the whole experience.

Many people don't get to hear that they are appreciated until it is too late, Brian got to hear it while he was still alive and I am sure this helped him hang on as long as he did. Getting a message from his idol Michael McDonald touched him deeply. Michael had sung on a song called Celebrate the Season in a duet with Andreas Aleman and it was a big deal for Brian to have him sing one of his songs.

Recovery

Recovery is a slow process. It is about learning patience every day. The importance of doing the little things today that will help you move towards tomorrow, and then the next day and the next.

Wanting to Die

It is very important to get permission from your family to let go. If the family brushes it away and doesn't listen to what lies behind those words they will cause more sorrow and anxiety in the person dying. Say yes, give permission to die and then talk about the things that matter most. After that conversation you will feel relief even if it causes sadness. Sometimes things change afterwards. In Brian's case he was able to come back and realize he still had things to live for and accomplish. He was not done yet.

The Healing Room, a Sanctuary

The importance of having a healing place, a safe space where you can open up and let your worries out. It does not have to be anything fancy, it can be that you dedicate your favorite corner in your house where you put a chair and anything else you want to surround yourself with. Let that place be where you let go of fear and where you gain insights and can re-energize yourself through visualization and meditation. Let people know how you feel and that you love them. Learn to live one day at a time because that is something we all have in common, just one day at a time.

Avoiding Negative People

When you are ill it is important to surround yourself with people who give you energy and to not take on other people's grief. Be cautious of what you take in and believe in. A hasty word by an oncologist can send you spiraling downwards. Be clear and set boundaries even when it means having to say no to visits from dear friends.

Limiting the input from the outer world through news, TV etc. is also helpful. Be mindful of everything you take in and how it affects your path to healing.

Fear

Fear is the number one emotion that can paralyze you and it is usually masked by other feelings like anger and worry. If you scratch the surface of those two you will most likely find fear underneath. That is why it is important to face your fears.

Brian was a sensitive soul and I think it reflects in many of his lyrics. On the other hand he never quite understood my spiritual path and the work I was doing as a therapist although he had always been supporting me 100 %. He used to say with a smile that this was his first incarnation and that was why he was so slow in catching up with me. As he got cancer this second time around he finally got it. The switch was amazing to see and he really caught up quickly and became very spiritual. I never thought we would have those deep conversations about the meaning and purpose of life and death. He was scared before and by avoiding the topic he thought he could avoid cancer coming back. I know he learned that you cannot sweep your fears under the rug and pretend they are not there. Sooner or later you have to face them full on and the longer you wait, the bigger they seem.

When it comes to fear it is one of our most fundamental drives to either run, fight or simply freeze. Fear can help us avoid or escape dangerous situations but it can also make us paralyzed. The fear of cancer is not something you can outrun. Trying to avoid dealing with it puts an enormous stress on the immune system and further lowers our chances of coming out alive. But what if you know that the chance of surviving a stage 4 metastasized cancer is low? To be able to have any kind of life quality at the end, this is one of the most important issues to deal with and not let fear take over your whole life. Brian showed it can be done.

The possibility of death is something most people avoid talking about and still the death rate is 100% for all of us.

By breaking fears down into smaller segments it makes them more manageable and by turning on the headlights and facing them straight on with someone else by your side makes it less scary.

Epilogue

*I*t didn't really start with the cancer diagnosis on July 17, 2017. His first cancer of the thyroid was operated in 2010 and they took out the whole thyroid and he never needed any other cancer treatments after that except for lifelong medication. In October 2015 he was hit with severe heart failure, arrhythmia and atrial fibrillation that got worse over the years even with medication. By June 2017 I did not dare to leave him alone at home in case something would happen so our sons and I, unbeknown to Brian, had a planned schedule so he would never be left alone. Brian had been waiting to get a new heart valve during 2017 but getting the operation was hard due to lack of staff at the hospital.

When I go back and look at my calendar from the beginning of June 2017, I can tell that even I was hit by severe tiredness and loss of energy. I had been working too much for too many years starting up a nonprofit organization and the lack of income was tough on both of us. I also had a deadline on a course that I was able to finish July 10, one week before Brian got his diagnosis. On July 17, the day of his diagnosis, we were supposed to take two weeks off before starting work again. I must have picked up his sickness energetically and could not understand why

I, who had never had headaches or problems sleeping, all of a sudden suffered from both.

On June 17, exactly one month before Brian's diagnosis, he really scared me. We had visitors from the States, one of Brian's oldest friends and his wife, and we took them to Drottningholm castle here in Stockholm for sightseeing. While visiting the old theater he became more and more quiet. I looked at Brian and he was white in his face and sweating. I took him outside in the fresh air and sat him under a tree in the shade while getting some water. His heart was beating irregularly, worse than ever before. Being as stubborn as he was, he did not want to go to the hospital so he just sat under a tree waiting for it to pass. On the following Monday morning we started pushing for new tests and trying to get his operation moved forward but with Midsummer and vacation times around the corner, we quickly learned that being sick in the summer is not optimal.

To cut a long story short, more tests were done and this time they also checked his blood. Something was not right. Brian had had constant heart problems during the whole year and finally on July 17 we went to see his cardiologist and instead of telling us about when he could get a new heart valve, we were told that Brian had a 12 centimeter large tumor on his left kidney and that it had already spread to the liver. Now we were faced with more than a heart problem.

On July 31 they removed his tumor and left kidney. Brian was living with a scenario that once the tumor was gone he would have a month of recuperating and then be able to go back to school as a teacher. For me this was the hardest time as I knew from the moment he got the diagnosis what it meant, but I did not want Brian to know the grim facts. It would have killed his spirit right away and I doubt it would have done him any good. He found out in time and it hit him hard.

Right from the start on July 17, which was supposed to be the start of our vacation, I decided to stay at home and help him through whatever happened. We started right away with a change in diet and focusing on his mental wellbeing and just prepping him to be strong for the surgery.

It turned out to be seven months focusing on one patient, my husband, and it was the most important thing I have done in my life. He asked me at one stage if I had learned something new during the experience and after much thinking I said no but that I was thankful to be able to be such a big part of his life during these difficult times. Brian on the other hand learned a lot and got to understand why I was so passionate about my work with cancer patients. Previously he never understood how I could work with something as depressing as counseling people with cancer but now he realized it was one of the most rewarding things to do.

During Brian's last month he no longer had the strength to write and he started his transition from doing to just being. He went deeper inside himself but at the same time needed us to be closer than ever. It was a time where just being there was enough, everything had been said and we had said our goodbyes plenty of times. I will never forget the stillness during the last hour in Brian's life before he left us. It was a peaceful hour and to be able to take that last trip we make once in our lifetime surrounded by family must be one of the best send-offs you can receive and the greatest gift you can give.

This book shows the ups and down, from hope to despair and back to hope, and that it can happen quickly and many times during a day. I wish it will give you strength to find your passion and to pursue it whether you are facing an illness or just feel stuck in your life.

It has been over a year since Brian passed away and life has changed dramatically. I am now, more than ever, convinced that by facing whatever fear you are challenged with, it will lead to greater peace of mind. Brian went peacefully on February 8, 2018 surrounded by family and our dog by his side.

Fia Hobbs

Benediction

The essence of our soul
Was never born and will never die
All we are is light
Experiencing a body
for a while

Divine sparks
Going home
To where we came from

Written by Fia Hobbs and it was read at Brian's memorial by Adam Hobbs.

Texts and Lyrics Brian Wrote during His Diagnosis

THIS SIDE OF THE DIRT

Chorus
Now I'm just tryin' to stay here
on this side of the dirt
Tryin' to find a way to get through
Another day of the hurt
Some days are better
and some days are worse
But I ain't down and I ain't gone
I'm holding on
To this side of the dirt

Verse
I used to take this life for granted
Forgot that all we have is time
Thought my life was somehow enchanted
It only happens to the other guy

Then I got that big old wake-up call
Told me I was just a man
And I was on my knees, my back against the wall
Praying give me one more chance

Pre
And I got thoughtful
And I got thankful
And I saw beauty where I'd never seen it before
Yes I got thoughtful
And I got thankful
For the pain and joy and love and so much more

DANCE ME INTO FOREVER

Dance me into forever
Past the nevermore
Past the closing doors
Dance me into forever
Past the railroad tracks
Past the looking back
And let me swirl through the starry, starry night
Through the rainbow sounds
Through the gardens of earthly delights
Make me change just like the weather
Dance me into forever

LOVE IS HERE

No one really knows how it all begins
That feeling that comes over you that you
never want to end
When all is glitter and light
And things you can't explain
When your arms are full of dreams
That you thought you'd thrown way

When you can suddenly see
Your doubts and fears unwind and disappear
And you know that finally, finally
Love is here

Deep inside yourself there's a secret place
And there amidst the emptiness
Is a chance you want to take
And … are treasures that shine
Where once you hid your pain
And the relics of your past
Are forgotten yesterdays

And you can suddenly see
Your doubts and fears unwind and disappear
And you know that finally
After all the intrigue
Unexpectedly the mysteries revealed
And you're here next to me and now it's all so clear, finally, maybe
     endlessly
Love is here

HOW MANY TIMES

How many times have you thought about time
The seasons that change and the yesterdays
You've left behind
How many times in the still of the night
Do you lie there awake
With your eyes open wide
How many times have you talked to the wind
And heard the willow tree sing through the rain
And how many times have you thought
About dreams and how you're still in mine

How many times have you looked at me
And just kept walking by

ALL THE THINGS I LOST

All the things I lost lie scattered across the scribbled pages of my life.
I see them, just out of reach, glistening like ornaments.
And the memories of these things, these times and people,
Fall apart like rain or snow, covering my face,
And I use them to hide my sorrow.

I flip through the empty pages of my future life,
The white, pristine paper offers so many possibilities,
And yet I feel trapped in the whiteness,
Wishing I had polished the script,
Wishing I and the other actors had remembered the lines,
Had not missed our marks.

All the things I lost haunt me and shine so much brighter than what I
   have.
And I hear the scratch of the pen and wonder if my story,
My being and future-time will be blinded by wanting the things I
   can't reach,
If my destiny consists of looking back but falling forward into the abyss
But these things are beautiful and they do make me smile sometimes.
And they glitter beautifully through my tears.

About Brian Hobbs

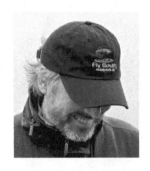

Brian Hobbs (1958-2018), was a songwriter originally from Elizabeth City, North Carolina and resided in Stockholm Sweden since 1992 with his wife Fia Hobbs and their twin boys. He attended the Berklee College of Music in Boston Massachusetts and worked as a songwriting teacher at Kulturama in Stockholm Sweden. While living in New York, besides working at the commodity exchange, he was a member of the ASCAP Musical Theater Workshop, the Lehman Engel BMI Musical Theater Workshop, the ASCAP POP music workshop and the ASCAP R&B music workshop. Once in Sweden, he was signed to MCA Music Publishing (now Universal) and was also a staff writer for Multiplay Music Ltd. based in London.

He has had songs recorded by and worked with a wide range of artists in Sweden such as Björn Skifs, Janne Schaffer, Jill Johnson, Monica Silverstrand, Mia Löfgren, Johan Becker, Andreas Aleman, Stefan Gunnarsson, Nils Landgren, Peter Getz, Victoria Tolstoy and many others. He has also had hits in Japan with groups like Arashi.

He has also had songs recorded by artists in Spain, Belgium, China, the Philippines, Portugal, Iceland, Norway, Denmark and in the US, including Michael McDonald, O.C. Smith and Joseph Williams of TOTO. He independently released albums by artists such as Andreas Aleman, *This is Life* (2009), *It's the Journey* (2012), *Home for Christmas* (2014) and Monica Silverstrand, *Been There, Done That* (2005).

Brian also released 7 albums under his own name; *Music for Balancing Body & Mind* (2001), *Impressions of the Outer Banks* (2003), *Candle in the Window* (2006), *Second Glances* (2010), *Genesis of Who I Am* (2017), *Reflections* (2017), the score to his musical, *The Independent Man* (2017) and *Love Remembered* (2012) with the Albert-Hobbs Big Band, *Impressions of the Outer Banks II* (2017), *Healing Purpose* (2018).

He published an eBook in 2018 called *The Craft of Creating* and this book is the culmination of his years of experience as a songwriter and producer and as a songwriting teacher in Stockholm, Sweden. The book *Reflections* is based on his blog during his illness and final months.

About Fia Hobbs

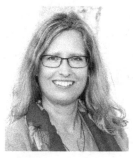

Fia Hobbs is born in Sweden and has lived in many different countries over the years. She is an international speaker and expert on stress management, counseling therapist, writer and founder of a non-profit organization in Sweden called Fonden CancerFriskvård (Foundation for Cancer Wellness).

She has been working in healthcare since 1989 and runs her company Arcadia FriskVård AB.

Brian came into her life in 1988 while she was working in New York and they got married a year later. She gave birth to their twin boys in 1992.

Aside from her work as a counseling therapist, her main focus has been stress management for the past 30 years including qigong, meditation, mindfulness and body treatments. She has a Master's degree in Medical Qigong and has done clinic work in China and Japan. Her training also includes assistant nursing and she had the privilege of studying under Dr Carl Simonton at the Simonton Cancer Center. She has also studied Cognitive Behavioral Therapy, (CBT) Neuro Linguistic Programming (NLP) and Motivational Interviewing (MI).

In 2010 she released her first book in Swedish called *East meets West: Mental Training Across the Divide* and in 2015 she co-wrote the book *Boosta din Business*, also in Swedish.